Pocket Diagnosis in General Surgery

D1396332

ST BARTHOLOMEW'S AND THE ROY
SCHOOL OF M

WHITE

Pocket Diagnosis in General Surgery

A companion to Lecture Notes on General Surgery

HAROLD ELLIS

CBE DM FRCS FRCOG
Emeritus Professor of Surgery
University of London
Department of Anatomy and Cell Biology
Guy's, King's and St Thomas'
School of Biomedical Sciences
London

CHRISTOPHER J.E. WATSON

MA MD FRCS
Lecturer in Surgery & Honorary Consultant
Department of Surgery
University of Cambridge
Addenbrooke's Hospital
Cambridge

Third Edition

b

Blackwell
Science

© 1990, 1993, 2001 by
Blackwell Science Ltd
Editorial Offices:
Osney Mead, Oxford OX2 0EL
25 John Street, London WC1N 2BS
23 Ainslie Place, Edinburgh EH3 6AJ
350 Main Street, Malden
  MA 02148-5018, USA
54 University Street, Carlton
  Victoria 3053, Australia
10, rue Casimir Delavigne
  75006 Paris, France

Other Editorial Offices:
Blackwell Wissenschafts-Verlag GmbH
Kurfürstendamm 57
10707 Berlin, Germany

Blackwell Science KK
MG Kodenmacho Building
7–10 Kodenmacho Nihombashi
Chuo-ku, Tokyo 104, Japan

Iowa State University Press
A Blackwell Science Company
2121 S. State Avenue
Ames, Iowa 50014-8300, USA

First published 1990
Second edition 1993
Third edition 2001

Set by Best-set Typesetter Ltd., Hong Kong
Printed and bound in Italy by
Rotolito Lombarda S.p.A., Milan

DISTRIBUTORS

  Marston Book Services Ltd
  PO Box 269
  Abingdon, Oxon OX14 4YN
  (*Orders*:   Tel: 01235 465500
              Fax: 01235 465555)

USA
  Blackwell Science, Inc.
  Commerce Place
  350 Main Street
  Malden, MA 02148-5018
  (*Orders*:   Tel: 800 759 6102
                    781 388 8250
              Fax: 781 388 8255)

Canada
  Login Brothers Book Company
  324 Saulteaux Crescent
  Winnipeg, Manitoba R3J 3T2
  (*Orders*:   Tel: 204 837 2987)

Australia
  Blackwell Science Pty Ltd
  54 University Street
  Carlton, Victoria 3053
  (*Orders*:   Tel: 3 9347 0300
              Fax: 3 9347 5001)

A catalogue record for this title
is available from the British Library

ISBN 0-632-05479-4

Library of Congress
Cataloging-in-publication Data
Ellis, Harold, 1926–
    Pocket diagnosis in general surgery : a
  companion to Lecture notes on general surgery /
  Harold Ellis, Christopher J.E. Watson.—3rd ed.
        p. ; cm.
    Includes index.
    ISBN 0-632-05479-4
    1. Surgery—Handbooks, manuals, etc.
  I. Watson, Christopher J. E. (Christopher John
  Edward) II. Ellis, Harold, 1926– . Lecture notes on
  general surgery. III. Title.
    [DNLM: 1. Surgical Procedures, Operative—
  Case Report. 2. Surgical Procedures, Operative—
  Examination Questions. 3. Surgical Procedures,
  Operative—Handbooks.
  WO 18.2 E47p 2000]
  RD37 .E44 2000
  617—dc21   00-067484

For further information on
Blackwell Science, visit our website:
www.blackwell-science.com

Contents

Foreword, vi

Preface, vii

Acknowledgements, viii

Questions, 1

Cases, 253

'In the foreword to the first edition of this book I suggested that a diagnostic quiz was a very good way of reinforcing vital clinical lessons. We are now in the third edition and Professor Harold Ellis has been joined by Mr Christopher Watson who is an experienced teacher and consultant general surgeon at Addenbrooke's Hospital, Cambridge. Between them they have improved the text and selection of pictures, which were already good in the first edition. Surgery moves quickly and diagnostic techniques and investigations are changing rapidly. These changes are reflected in this volume which I am confident will be as popular and successful as the earlier editions.

Sir Roy Calne

Lecture Notes on General Surgery presents most of the factual material required by final year medical students who are approaching their qualifying examinations. This collection of photographs of patients, of pathological specimens, of X-rays and of CT scans supplements this text. We believe it will provide excellent practise for the skills which the student needs to display in the oral and 'short case' parts of Finals in Surgery.

The questions follow sequentially the chapters in *Lecture Notes* and the answers are based on its text.

The need for a third edition has enabled us to revise and update the text, to add a number of new 'spots' and to include a number of case studies.

It is hoped that this book will be as helpful in assisting medical students through the hurdles of their qualifying examination as its sister volume has proved to be in the past.

Harold Ellis, London
Christopher Watson, Cambridge
2001

Acknowledgements

We owe a deep debt of gratitude to the staff of the Medical Photographic Department at Westminster Hospital and Addenbrooke's Hospital who provided the great bulk of the illustrations as well as skilled technical advice. The staff of the Department of Radiology at Westminster Hospital and Addenbrooke's Hospital were most helpful in assisting with the selection of suitable X-rays and CT scans. We would like to thank a number of colleagues for the loan of specialist illustrations — Mr Paul Aichroth (orthopaedics), Dr A. Branfoot (pathology) and Mr D. Forrest and Professor L. Spitz (paediatrics).

We are grateful to our co-author of *Lecture Notes on General Surgery*, Professor Sir Roy Calne FRS, for his generous foreword.

Finally, we would like to thank the staff of Blackwell Science for the difficult task of seeing this book through its production.

QUESTIONS

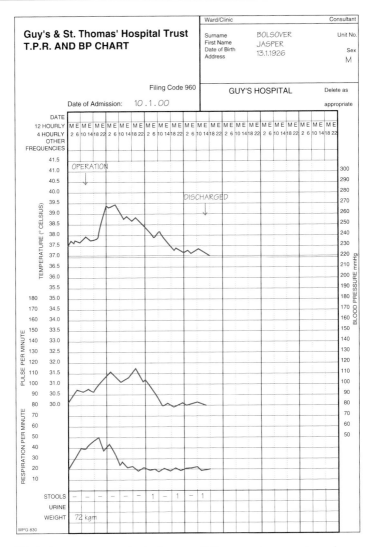

This is the temperature chart of a man of 75 years, a heavy smoker, who required emergency surgery for a strangulated right inguinal hernia. After a rather stormy post-operative period, he recovered.

1 What is the most likely cause of this post-operative pyrexia?

2 What causes this complication?

3 What factors were probably responsible in this particular patient?

4 What physical signs of this complication would you have expected to find when you examined this patient on the first post-operative day?

5 How was he (successfully) treated?

1 Post-operative pulmonary collapse.

2 Mucus retention in the bronchial tree.

3 (a) *Pre-operative factor*: heavy cigarette smokers often have chronic bronchitis.

(b) *Operative factor*: the irritation of anaesthetic drugs.

(c) *Post-operative factor*: the pain of the groin incision would inhibit expectoration of the accumulated bronchial secretions.

4 The patient would be dyspnoeic with a rapid pulse and elevated temperature. There may have been cyanosis. He would have a painful 'fruity' cough. Chest movements would be diminished with basal dullness, depressed air entry and the presence of crackles.

5 Vigorous breathing exercises and encouragement to cough, assisted by repeated doses of morphia. In his case, as the sputum was mucopurulent, ampicillin was also prescribed.

(See Chapter 3, *Lecture Notes on General Surgery*.)

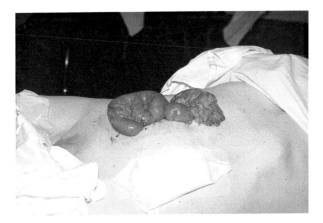

This patient coughed 10 days after his gastrectomy and called the nurses to see this frightening sight.

1 What is this condition called?

2 What may be a warning sign that this is to happen?

3 How would you classify the factors that may be responsible for this emergency?

4 If you were the House Surgeon on duty, what would be your immediate emergency steps in dealing with this?

5 If the deep layers of the incision give way but the skin holds intact, what will result?

1 Burst abdomen (dehiscence of the abdominal wound).

2 The 'pink fluid sign' — serous blood-tinged fluid may ooze through the wound for a day or two before the actual burst occurs.

3 The aetiology of any post-operative complication should be thought of under the headings of pre-operative, operative and post-operative factors. In this case, *pre-operative factors* include anything that affects wound healing, such as uraemia, protein deficiency, vitamin C deficiency or chronic cough. At *operation*, poor technique, and *post-operative*, cough or abdominal distension, wound infection or wound haematoma.

4 Reassure the patient (he would be terrified), give opiate analgesia, cover the exposed bowel with saline-soaked sterile dressing and arrange transfer to the operating theatre for immediate re-suture.

5 An incisional hernia.

(See Chapter 3, *Lecture Notes on General Surgery*.)

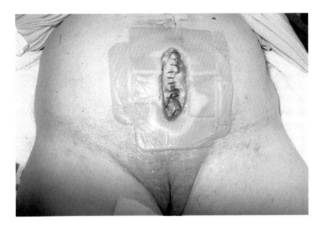

This patient discharged faecal fluid and flatus through the lower end of her wound after resection of a recto-sigmoid carcinoma.

1 What is this condition called?

2 What is the definition of this term?

3 What is the sheet surrounding the wound called, and what is its importance?

4 How can the track be visualized radiologically?

5 In general terms, what might prevent such a lesion from healing spontaneously?

1 Post-operative faecal fistula.

2 A fistula is a pathological track that connects two epithelial surfaces (in this case, colon and skin).

3 Stomahesive; this adheres even to moist skin. A collecting bag is attached to this, thus preventing enzyme-containing effluent from reaching (and digesting) the skin around the fistula.

4 By X-raying the patient after injection of radio-opaque contrast (e.g. Gastrograffin) through the fistula — 'a fistulogram'.

5 (a) Loss of continuity between the ends of the bowel.

   (b) Distal obstruction.

   (c) The presence of diseased tissue in the fistulous track.

(See Chapter 3, *Lecture Notes on General Surgery*.)

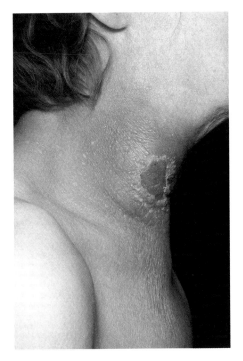

This 55-year-old woman developed this lesion following a scratch on the neck.

1 What is this called?
2 What does this term mean?
3 What are its characteristic physical features?
4 What is the commonest organism to produce this?
5 How is it treated?

1 Cellulitis.

2 A spreading infection of connective tissues.

3 The four characteristics of inflammation—heat, redness, swelling and pain. There may be blistering of the overlying skin and, in severe cases, cutaneous gangrene.

4 The beta haemolytic streptococcus.

5 Where possible (e.g. a limb) immobilization. Penicillin (or erythromycin in allergic patients).

(See Chapter 4, *Lecture Notes on General Surgery*.)

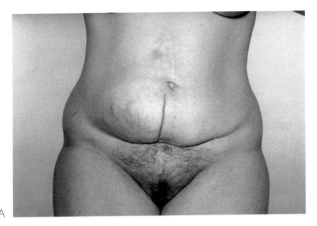

A

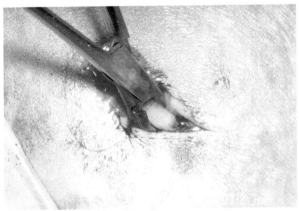

B

This 42-year-old woman was admitted as an emergency. A few weeks previously she had a benign ovarian cyst removed at laparotomy. She now presents with a large abscess in the subcutaneous tissues of the lower right abdomen (A). The surgical procedure she underwent later that day is shown in (B).

1 What is the definition of an abscess?
2 What general manifestations often accompany this?
3 What procedure is being performed in (B)?
4 What would have happened if this had not been carried out?
5 What should be the post-operative management of this patient?

1 An abscess is a localized collection of pus, usually, but not invariably, produced by pyogenic organisms.

2 Associated features may be a swinging temperature, malaise, anorexia and sweating with a polymorph leucocytosis.

3 The abscess is being drained through a small incision. The track has been widened by means of forceps inserted through the wound and the pus is being evacuated.

4 If not drained, the abscess would eventually discharge, probably through the recent abdominal wound. However, during this time the pus would continue to act as a source of toxaemia and the patient would remain extremely ill.

5 Drainage is maintained until the abscess cavity heals from below upwards. This is achieved by means of inserting a gauze wick, a corrugated drain or a tube. The drain is gradually withdrawn until complete healing is achieved.

(See Chapter 4, *Lecture Notes on General Surgery*.)

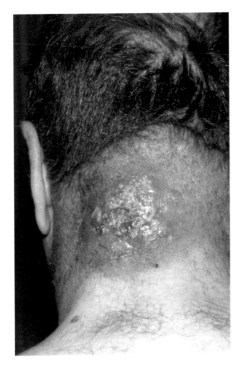

This man, aged 58, came to casualty with this unpleasant lesion on his neck, which had been present for several days.

1 What is it called?

2 What is the definition of this lesion?

3 What simple investigation should be carried out in the casualty department for a possible underlying cause?

4 What is the usual organism causing this condition?

5 How is it treated?

1 A carbuncle.

2 An area of subcutaneous necrosis, which discharges onto the surface through multiple sinuses; it is these multiple sinuses that give this characteristic appearance.

3 Test the urine for sugar and, if positive, perform a confirmatory blood sugar estimation. Always think of diabetes in septic conditions such as this.

4 Almost invariably *Staphylococcus aureus* — this can be checked by bacteriological examination of a smear of the pus.

5 Antibiotic therapy — flucloxacillin (or erythromycin if penicillin-sensitive).

(See Chapter 4, *Lecture Notes on General Surgery*.)

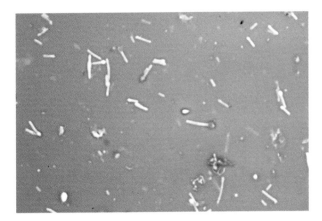

This smear of a bacterial culture shows characteristic terminal 'drum stick' spores on Gram-positive rods.

1 What is this organism?
2 What is its normal habitat?
3 What is the type of toxin it produces and what are its effects?
4 Is it an anaerobic or aerobic organism — and why is this important?
5 List the effective prophylactic measures against infection by this organism.

1 *Clostridium tetani.*

2 This is a normal inhabitant of soil and faeces.

3 An exotoxin, which acts upon the motor cells in the CNS.

4 The bacterium is anaerobic and tetanus may therefore follow implantation of this organism into devitalized tissues where anaerobic conditions occur.

5 Active immunization—tetanus toxoid (formalin-treated exotoxin), two initial injections at an interval of 6 weeks. Booster doses at intervals of not more than 7 years or at the time of any injury. Passive prophylaxis comprises adequate excision of contaminated wounds to remove all dead tissue, prophylactic penicillin and a booster dose of toxoid in patients who have previously been immunized. If toxoid has not been given in the past, human gamma globulin, prepared from fully immunized subjects, should be given if the wound is heavily contaminated.

(See Chapter 4, *Lecture Notes on General Surgery.*)

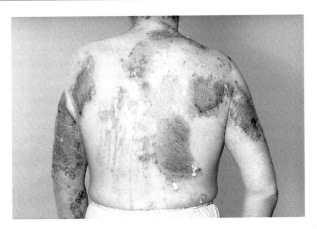

This patient burnt the back of his chest and his upper arms at work. This photograph was taken 10 days after the accident.

1 How deep are these burns?

2 What further treatment will probably be needed for the burns on his arms and over his right scapula?

3 Roughly, what area of his body surface has been affected?

4 Why is estimation of the area of the burn of value in management?

5 What local treatment would you have given to these burns?

1 The burns over most of the back are partial thickness. The underlying germinal layer is intact and healing is taking place. The burns on the arms and on the right shoulder are full thickness. The overlying coagulum is adherent to underlying granulation tissue.

2 These full-thickness burns were excised the following day and covered with split skin grafts taken from the thigh.

3 Approximately 14%. About half of the back of the trunk has been involved — roughly 9% — and using the patient's hand as representing 1% of the body surface, the burns on the arms represent another 5%.

4 The severity of the burn and the amount of fluid loss from the burn is proportional to the surface area of the burn.

5 This could be treated by the closed technique using silver sulphadiazine (Flamazine) covered by thick layers of sterile dressings. In fact, as only the posterior aspect of the patient was burnt, the open (or exposure) method was used.

(See Chapter 6, *Lecture Notes on General Surgery*.)

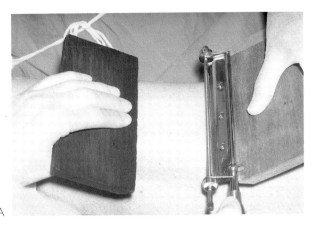

A

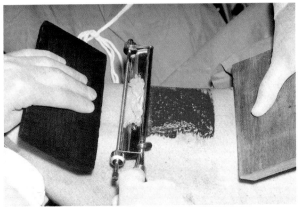

B

(A) and (B) represent two stages of an operation on this patient's thigh. He had sustained severe burns to his hands and face a week previously.

1 What operation is being performed?

2 What layers of skin are being removed by the surgeon?

3 What will happen to the raw area left behind on the patient's thigh?

4 What are the priority areas for skin grafting in a patient with extensive full-thickness burns?

1 Skin is being taken for a skin graft.

2 This is a 'split skin' graft taken through the germinal layer of the epithelium and leaving islands of this layer at the donor site.

3 The remaining islands of germinal epithelium in the donor site will proliferate so that the raw area will become re-epithelialized in about 10 days.

4 The eyelids have top priority, followed by face, hands and the flexor aspects of the joints. These are the situations where scarring would produce considerable deformity and disability.

(See Chapter 6, *Lecture Notes on General Surgery*.)

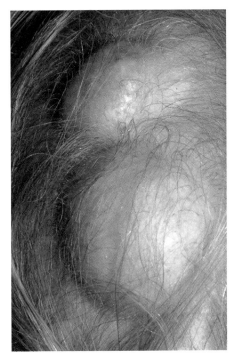

This woman presented with these mobile cystic masses in the scalp.

1 What is the diagnosis?

2 Where else are they commonly found, and where on the skin do they *never* occur?

3 What do they look like when excised and cut open?

4 What complications may they undergo?

5 How should they be treated?

1 Sebaceous cysts of the scalp.

2 Apart from the scalp, which is the commonest site, they are found frequently on the face, scrotum, vulva and the lobule of the ear. They are *not* found on the gland-free palms and soles.

3 There is a white lining membrane of squamous epithelium. The contents are cheesy with an unpleasant smell.

4 (a) Infection.
   (b) Ulceration ('Cock's peculiar tumour').
   (c) Calcification.
   (d) Horn formation.
   (e) Malignant change.

5 Because of the risk of infection, patients should always be advised to have their sebaceous cysts excised. This can be done quite simply under local anaesthetic. If acutely inflamed, drainage will be required, followed later by excision of the capsule wall.

(See Chapter 7, *Lecture Notes on General Surgery*.)

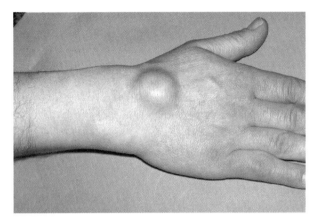

This patient presented with a painless cystic swelling on the wrist, which had gradually enlarged over the past year.

1 What is your clinical diagnosis?
2 Where else are these cysts commonly found?
3 What are the theories of their origin?
4 What material do they contain?
5 What is the prognosis following surgical excision?

1 Ganglion of the wrist.

2 The dorsum of the foot (arising from joint capsule), on the flexor sheaths of the fingers and on the peroneal tendon sheaths.

3 They may represent a benign myxoma of a joint capsule or tendon sheath, a hamartoma or a myxomatous degeneration of the joint capsule or tendon sheath due to trauma.

4 Mucoid fluid having the microscopic appearances of Wharton's jelly.

5 Recurrence is unfortunately quite common after surgical excision if even a fragment of the ganglion wall is left behind.

(See Chapter 7, *Lecture Notes on General Surgery*.)

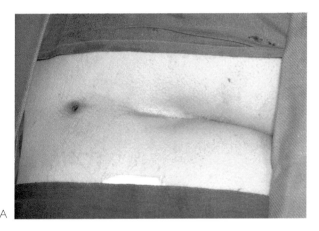

A

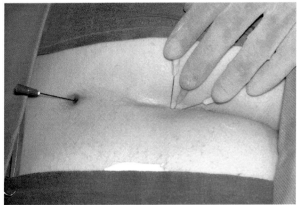

B

This is the sacral region of a young man about to undergo surgery (A). In (B), probes have been placed into three small orifices just above the anal verge and into the larger, more distal, opening of a discharging abscess.

1 What is the diagnosis?
2 What does this term mean?
3 What is the definition of a sinus?
4 What is the probable aetiology of this disease?
5 What type of patient characteristically develops this condition?

1 Pilonidal sinus with an associated abscess.

2 'Pilonidal' means a nest of hair.

3 A sinus is a blind track leading to a surface.

4 Implantation of hair into the skin sets up a foreign body reaction and produces a chronic infected sinus.

5 Young adults, males much more commonly than females, and particularly in dark-haired individuals. Barbers may develop pilonidal sinuses between their fingers.

(See Chapter 7, *Lecture Notes on General Surgery*.)

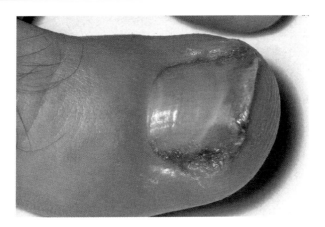

This patient has two lesions affecting his hallux, one of which has resulted in the other.

I What is the underlying lesion?

2 What is the secondary inflammatory process called?

3 How could the infection have been prevented?

4 How should the infection be treated in the acute phase?

5 What treatment may be needed in recurrent cases?

1 Ingrowing toenail.

2 Paronychia.

3 Avoid cutting the nail downwards into the nail fold, avoid tight shoes, tuck a pledget of cotton wool daily into the side of the nail bed to enable the nail to grow up out of the fold.

4 Drainage of the pus by removal of the side of the nail or avulsion of the whole nail.

5 The nail should be obliterated, either by excision of the nail root (Zadek's operation) or by treating the nail bed with phenol.

(See Chapter 7, *Lecture Notes on General Surgery*.)

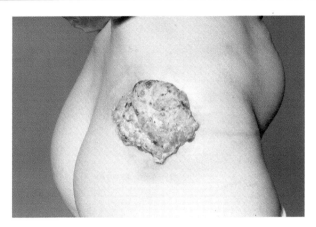

This woman, aged 55, completely neglected this mass over her right hip for several years until it reached this size. By this time she already had a cluster of hard, enlarged lymph nodes in the right groin.

1 What would be your clinical diagnosis?

2 This is a relatively unusual site for this tumour. Where is it more often found?

3 What are the predisposing factors for the development of this tumour?

4 Left untreated, what would be the likely cause of death of this woman?

5 How was this patient treated?

1 This is likely to be a squamous carcinoma of the skin with lymphatic metastases. (This was confirmed on biopsy.)

2 Squamous carcinoma of the skin usually occurs on areas exposed to sunshine, e.g. the face and on the backs of the hands.

3 Predisposing factors include exposure to sunshine or irradiation, exposure to carcinogens (e.g. pitch, tar and soot), malignant change in senile keratosis, lupus vulgaris and chronic ulcers (Marjolin's ulcer), malignant change in Bowen's disease (carcinoma *in situ*) and, occasionally, in patients on long-term immuno-suppressive drugs.

4 Distant blood-borne metastases are not common. Death occurs from repeated haemorrhages, either from the untreated ulcerated primary tumour or from ulceration of the involved lymph nodes infiltrating the groin vessels.

5 Wide excision of the primary tumour with skin grafting followed by block dissection of the nodes in the groin. She achieved long-term survival!

(See Chapter 7, *Lecture Notes on General Surgery*.)

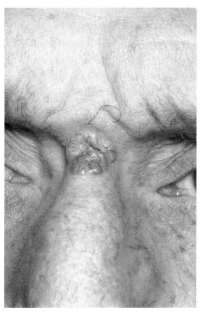

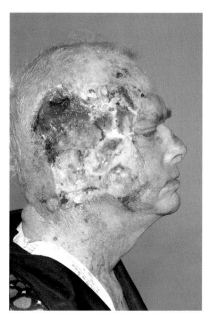

A   B

These two photographs represent patients with early (A) and late (B) examples of the same skin tumour.

1 What is the scientific name and the 'popular' name for this skin cancer?

2 What is the typical cutaneous distribution of this tumour?

3 What is its microscopic appearance?

4 How does it spread?

5 How may these tumours be treated?

1 Basal cell carcinoma or rodent ulcer.

2 90% are found on the face above a line joining the angle of the mouth to the external auditory meatus. It is especially common around the eye, the naso-labial folds and the hairline of the scalp.

3 Under the microscope, solid sheets of uniform, darkly staining cells are seen, which arise from the basal layer of the epidermis. Prickle cells and epithelial pearls (typical of squamous cell carcinoma) are both absent.

4 Spread is by slow but steady infiltration of surrounding tissues, which may include the underlying skull and meninges, face, nose and eye (hence the term 'rodent'). Lymphatic and blood spread are both extremely rare.

5 A small basal cell tumour can be treated by excision, where this can be done with an adequate margin and without cosmetic deformity. It may also be indicated in late cases, where the tumour has recurred after irradiation or has invaded underlying bone or cartilage. In these cases, major plastic surgical reconstruction may be necessary. In the majority of patients the lesion is treated by radiotherapy after biopsy confirmation of the diagnosis.

(See Chapter 7, *Lecture Notes on General Surgery*.)

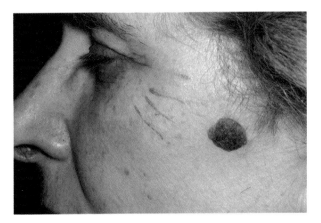

This woman has had this pigmented lesion ever since she can remember. It has not changed at all in size but she has now asked to have it removed for cosmetic reasons.

1 How frequent are benign melanomas in the white population?

2 What is their cutaneous distribution?

3 This lesion was excised and proved to be an intradermal melanoma — what does this term mean?

4 What is meant by a junctional melanoma?

5 When should pigmented lesions of the skin be removed?

1 Nearly every white person possesses one or more benign melanomas, commonly called moles.

2 The intradermal melanoma may be found in every situation except the palm of the hand, the sole of the foot or the scrotal skin, whereas the junctional melanoma may be found in any part of the skin surface.

3 An intradermal melanoma is situated entirely in the dermis, where melanocytes form non-encapsulated masses.

4 In contrast, the junctional melanoma shows melanocytes clumping together in the basal layer of the epidermis (i.e. the junction between the epidermis and dermis). It is the junctional naevus which may, in a small percentage of cases, undergo malignant change.

5 Excision of a pigmented skin lesion should be carried out:

(a) If the patient is worried about it or if it is cosmetically unpleasant.

(b) If it is situated on the hand, the sole or the genitalia.

(c) If the lesion shows any of the features that suggest that malignant change might have taken place (see Question 17).

(See Chapter 7, *Lecture Notes on General Surgery*.)

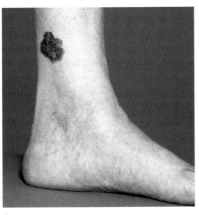

A

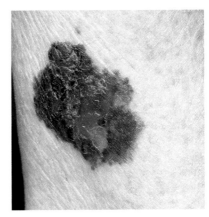

B

This young woman presented with a pigmented lesion above the ankle (A). It had been present for many years but in recent months it had enlarged quite rapidly. (B) is a closer view of the lesion.

1 What features suggest that this is a malignant melanoma?

2 What other local features (not present in her case) might suggest this diagnosis?

3 Where would you examine this patient next for evidence of metastatic spread?

4 Where else, apart from the skin, may malignant melanoma occur?

5 What factors will determine the prognosis in this case?

1 The history of recent enlargement is important. The melanoma shows irregularity in its outline and in its pigmentation — both highly suspicious.

2 Other local signs of malignant change are: bleeding or ulceration, spread of pigment from the edge of the tumour and surrounding daughter nodules. A history of itching or pain is also suspicious.

3 Carefully examine the ipsilateral inguinal nodes for enlargement.

4 Malignant melanoma may also be found on the mucous membrane of the nose, mouth, anal canal and intestine. In the eye, malignant melanoma may be found in the conjunctiva, the choroid and the pigmented layer of the retina.

5 Prognosis depends on:

(a) The thickness of the primary lesion. Prognosis is good when this is less than 1.5 mm in depth. The deeper the lesion, the greater the risk of lymph node spread.

(b) A superficial spreading melanoma has a better prognosis that a penetrating and ulcerating lesion.

(c) Tumours on the limbs have a better prognosis than those on the trunk and scalp.

(d) The presence of cutaneous deposits or lymph node metastases greatly increase the gravity of the prognosis, while blood-borne metastases (e.g. to liver) make the prognosis virtually hopeless.

(See Chapter 7, *Lecture Notes on General Surgery*.)

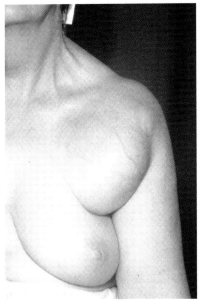

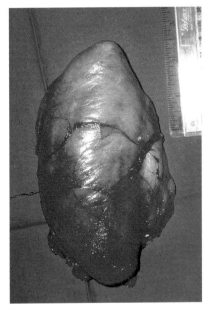

A

B

This woman presented with a very slowly enlarging subcutaneous mass on the left chest wall (A). The enucleated specimen is shown in (B).

1 What is the likely diagnosis?

2 What physical signs would you have expected to find on examining this lump?

3 Why did it fluctuate?

4 There are some subcutaneous areas where these tumours are *never* found — name them and explain why they are exempt.

5 Very rarely these tumours are malignant. What would suggest this clinically?

1 A lipoma.

2 A soft lobulated fluctuant swelling, not attached to the skin or underlying muscle. Transillumination would be positive.

3 A lipoma fluctuates because it is made up of aggregates of fat cells, each cell forming a microscopic cyst (fat is *not* liquid at body temperature).

4 Lipomas do not occur on the palm, the sole of the foot or the scalp because in these areas the fat is contained within dense fibrous septa.

5 A liposarcoma would be suggested if the tumour were rapidly growing, firmer than usual and vascular.

(See Chapter 7, *Lecture Notes on General Surgery*.)

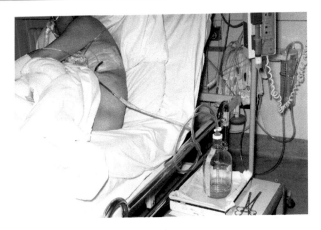

This patient has just undergone a thoracotomy.

1 What type of drain system is shown in this photograph?

2 How does this evacuate air from the pleural cavity?

3 How is air prevented from being sucked into the chest?

4 What precautions must be taken in positioning the water bottle?

5 Name two emergency situations when the insertion of such a tube in the Accident and Emergency Department could be life-saving.

1 An underwater chest drain.

2 Air is forced out through the water trap in the bottle during expiration.

3 Air cannot be sucked into the chest in inspiration—this is prevented by the water seal.

4 The bottle must be kept below the level of the chest, otherwise fluid may siphon back into the pleural cavity.

5 Tension pneumothorax; traumatic haemothorax.

(See Chapter 8, *Lecture Notes on General Surgery*.)

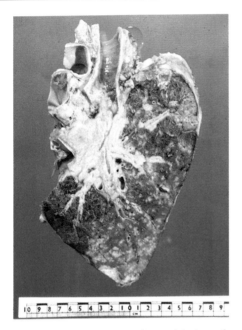

This is the post-mortem specimen of the lung of a man aged 68 years.

1 What is the obvious pathology?

2 About how many deaths are attributed to this disease annually in England and Wales?

3 What are the known predisposing factors?

4 List the main histological types of this condition.

5 List its pathways of spread.

1 Carcinoma of the lung.

2 40 000 deaths a year in England and Wales.

3 The main predisposing factor is smoking of cigarettes. Other factors are pollution of the air with diesel, petrol and other fumes. Radioactive carcinogens in certain mines are associated with carcinoma of the lung. The incidence is higher in urban than in rural populations.

4 40% squamous cell, 15% adenocarcinoma, 45% undifferentiated (either large polygonal cells or small elongated 'oat' cells).

5 (a) *Local* spread.
   (b) *Lymphatic* to mediastinal and cervical nodes.
   (c) *Blood* to bone, brain, liver, etc.
   (d) *Transcoelomic*, pleural seedlings and effusion.

(See Chapter 8, *Lecture Notes on General Surgery*.)

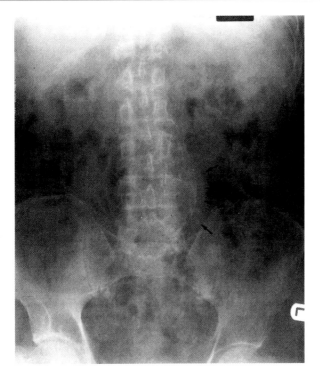

This patient, aged 70 years, was found to have a pulsating mass in his abdomen on routine examination. He was symptomless.

1 What does his abdominal X-ray show?
2 What other non-invasive imaging techniques can be used to demonstrate this lesion?
3 What is the principal danger of this condition?
4 What is the mortality of this complication?
5 How should this patient be managed?

1 The calcified wall of his abdominal aortic aneurysm (arrowed). Note that, as usually happens, it bulges over to the left side, away from the adjacent inferior vena cava.

2 CT scan or ultrasound; the latter is more often available and accessible.

3 Rupture — first retroperitoneally and then into the peritoneal cavity.

4 In the region of 80%.

5 Elective surgery with graft replacement.

(See Chapter 10, *Lecture Notes on General Surgery*.)

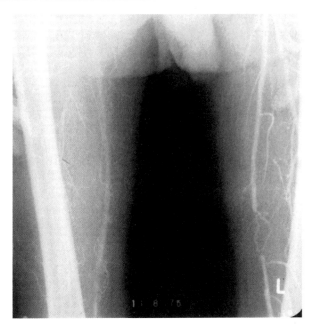

This is the arteriogram of a heavy smoker, aged 48, who complained of severe pain in the left calf on walking just a few yards. Fortunately, the skin of his foot is intact.

1 What does the arteriogram demonstrate?

2 Is an arteriogram performed routinely in all patients with claudication?

3 What is the condition of the artery distal to the obstruction — and why is this important?

4 What physical signs would you expect to find on examining this patient's left leg?

5 How can this patient's disabling symptoms be treated?

1 There is a short block in the superficial femoral artery on the left side. The main vessels show slight irregularity due to atherosclerosis.

2 No; arteriography is only performed if reconstructive surgery or balloon angioplasty is contemplated.

3 The distal superficial femoral artery and the popliteal artery are patent — this means that there is a good 'run off' and the patient is suitable for some form of reconstructive surgery.

4 The left foot is likely to be pale and cold. Buerger's sign will be positive. The pulses distal to the femoral pulse will almost certainly be absent. The return of capillary circulation after blanching the skin on the toes will be delayed. There may be guttering of the veins of the leg, especially when the leg is elevated.

5 Smoking must be prohibited. There is little point in performing any reconstructive surgery unless the patient gives up smoking because of the high risk of re-occlusion. This short section of obstruction could be treated either by open endarterectomy with a vein patch, or by angioplasty using a balloon catheter under X-ray control.

(See Chapter 10, *Lecture Notes on General Surgery*.)

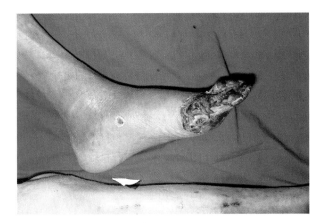

This 78-year-old man presented with rest pain in both legs and gangrene of the toes of the right foot. He is a heavy smoker and is also a diabetic.

1 What factors in diabetes contribute towards the gangrene?
2 What factors in smoking contribute towards this lesion?
3 What radiological investigation is indicated?
4 How may it be possible to save this patient's right leg?
5 What is the usual cause of death in patients such as this?

1 Diabetic micro-angiography, diabetic neuropathy and increased predisposition to infection.

2 Nicotine produces vasospasm, inhaled carbon monoxide in the smoke is taken up by the haemoglobin to form carboxyhaemoglobin, which reduces the oxygen-carrying capacity of the blood, and smoking increases platelet adhesiveness.

3 An arteriogram to determine whether or not reconstructive surgery is possible.

4 If a 'run off' is demonstrated, blood supply to the leg may be restored by reconstructive surgery or an angioplasty, hopefully with loss of only the gangrenous toes.

5 These patients usually succumb to the other complications of atherosclerosis—myocardial infarction, cardiac failure or stroke.

(See Chapter 10, *Lecture Notes on General Surgery*.)

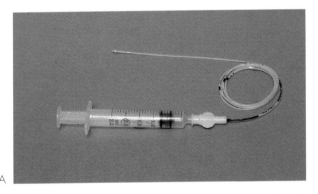

A

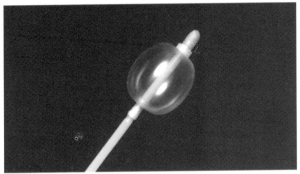

B

This is an important instrument used in vascular surgery; (B) is a close-up of its inflated tip.

1 What is it called?

2 What was the status of the inventor when he designed it?

3 What vascular emergency is it used for?

4 What treatment should be commenced when the patient is admitted with this emergency?

5 What is the most important factor that decides the prognosis of the limb in such a case?

1 A Fogarty catheter.

2 Thomas Fogarty thought of this as a clinical student and his reputation was made by the time he was a surgical resident.

3 Its principal use is to remove an occluding embolus and propagated clot from a blocked peripheral artery. It is slid down the artery through a proximal arteriotomy, the balloon inflated and the catheter withdrawn, allowing the embolus to be evacuated.

4 Intravenous heparin should be commenced at once to prevent further propagation of clot.

5 The likelihood of success of embolectomy is inversely proportional to the time interval from the onset of the block to the operation. After 24 hours have elapsed, successful disobliteration becomes less likely.

(See Chapter 10, *Lecture Notes on General Surgery*.)

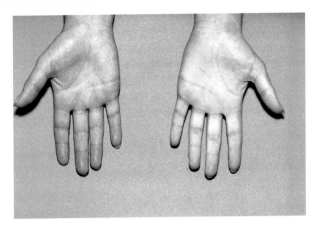

These are the hands of a woman, aged 20, on a warm summer's day. The left hand has just been placed in a bowl of cold water for 5 minutes.

1 What do you notice about the appearance of the left hand?
2 What disease would you suspect she has?
3 What are the typical clinical features of this condition?
4 What other conditions produce arterial impairment in the upper limb?
5 What treatment can be advised for this patient?

1 The left hand has become bluish-white compared with the normal pink appearance of the right hand.

2 Raynaud's disease.

3 Cold, painful hands (and often feet) dating back to childhood. The extremities become bluish-white in cold weather. Gangrene of the digital tips may rarely occur.

4 Atherosclerosis, cervical rib, scleroderma and other collagen diseases, cryoglobulinaemia and in workers using vibrating tools.

5 Conservative treatment includes the use of gloves and fur-lined boots and a trial of vasodilator drugs. Sympathectomy produces dramatic improvement but may not be long lasting in the upper limbs.

(See Chapter 10, *Lecture Notes on General Surgery*.)

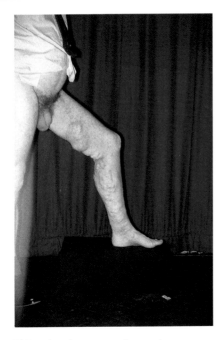

This patient has gross varicose veins.

1 What complication of this condition can you see affecting the varices in his thigh?

2 How should this complication be treated?

3 If you see a teenager with varicose veins, what would you usually find in the family history?

4 This patient has a particularly large bulge at the saphenous termination at the groin; what is this called?

5 If traumatized, varicose veins bleed copiously. How would you treat this emergency?

1 Acute phlebitis.

2 Bed rest, elevation of the leg. Antibiotics are rarely indicated as this is usually a sterile inflammatory process.

3 One or both parents and often siblings are also affected.

4 Saphena varix.

5 Lie the patient flat, elevate the leg (to reduce the venous pressure) and apply a pressure dressing.

(See Chapter 11, *Lecture Notes on General Surgery*.)

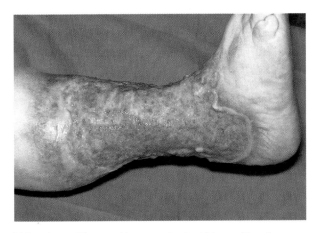

This patient, a 70-year-old woman, has had this condition for many years.

1 What names are given to it?

2 She has no evidence of varicose veins, so what is the likely aetiology of this problem?

3 What is a rare complication in long-standing cases?

4 What percentage of all leg ulcers in this country are venous in origin?

5 How would you treat this patient?

1 Varicose or gravitational ulcer.

2 A preceding deep venous thrombosis.

3 Malignant change — Marjolin's ulcer.

4 About 90%.

5 Elevate the leg whenever possible, Elastoplast bandaging over a paste bandage dressing, split skin graft of the ulcer if it remains indolent. Elastic stocking support once the ulcer has healed.

(See Chapter 11, *Lecture Notes on General Surgery*.)

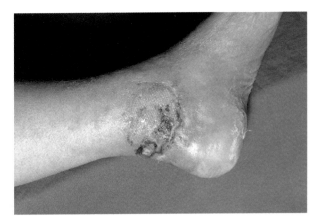

This elderly woman's ulcer had been treated for many months by conventional bandaging. When she was referred to hospital, the feet were found to be cold and blue and no pulses could be felt on either side below the femorals.

1 What is the diagnosis?
2 What symptom is she likely to experience on walking?
3 How can a Doppler ultrasonic probe be used to confirm the diagnosis?
4 List some of the other rarer causes of leg ulceration.

1 Ischaemic ulcer due to atherosclerosis.

2 Calf claudication.

3 Used in conjunction with a sphygmomanometer to compare the arm blood pressure with that obtained in the leg. There will be a considerable lowering of the ankle pressure compared with the brachial pressure.

4 Malignant ulcer, gumma, diabetes, an ulcer complicating other medical conditions such as ulcerative colitis, and self-inflicted injury.

(See Chapter 10, *Lecture Notes on General Surgery*.)

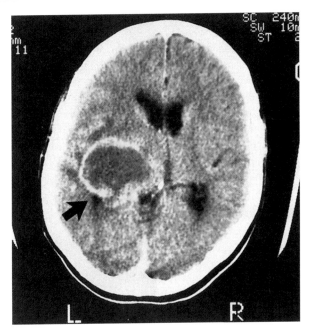

This is the CT scan, taken after an intravenous injection of enhancing material, of a young man who complained of increasingly severe headache of recent origin. Marked papilloedema was noted on fundal examination.

1 Describe the lesion which has been arrowed.

2 What effect is this having on the ventricular system?

3 A needle biopsy confirmed that this was a poorly differentiated astrocytoma — from which cells does this tumour arise, and what proportion of brain tumours does it comprise?

4 Where does this tumour occur typically in children?

5 What treatment is available for this patient, and what is the outlook for him?

1 There is an irregular cystic cavity with an intramural nodule. The wall of the cyst and the intramural nodule have taken up the contrast material. The mass arises in the left basal ganglia region and extends into the temporo-parietal lobe. The lesion is solitary. This is in favour of a primary tumour, since metastases in the brain are usually multiple.

2 The third ventricle is shifted to the right.

3 Gliomas arise from the glial supporting cells. Gliomas account for some 45% of intracranial tumours encountered in neurosurgical units. Secondary deposits in the brain are the commonest CNS tumours overall, but patients with widespread metastases do not usually come under neurosurgical care.

4 Cerebellum.

5 Palliative radiotherapy, which may be combined with surgical decompression. The prognosis is extremely bad in these poorly differentiated tumours.

(See Chapter 12, *Lecture Notes on General Surgery*.)

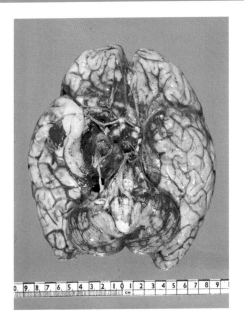

This is the brain of a previously healthy man of 40, who suddenly became co-matose and died a few days later.

1 Describe the pathological findings.
2 What is the commonest cause of the underlying lesion?
3 What other disease processes may produce this?
4 What is the natural history of this disease?
5 Outline the management of this condition.

1 There is a large right-sided aneurysm of the circle of Willis, which has ruptured. There is blood in the subarachnoid space.

2 95% of intracranial aneurysms are congenital.

3 Other causes are arteriosclerosis, trauma or infection (mycotic aneurysms).

4 A quarter of the patients with haemorrhage from a ruptured aneurysm die
without recovering consciousness, as in this case. More than 50% will bleed
again within 6 weeks of the initial haemorrhage and the mortality of such bleeds
is high. After 6 weeks the likelihood of haemorrhage becomes less but is still
present.

5 When the patient is in coma or has a dense hemiplegia, nursing care only is
indicated. If the patient recovers from the initial bleed, cerebral angiography
is performed to locate the site of the aneurysm before the peak
incidence of recurrent haemorrhage, which is after about 2 weeks. If an
aneurysm is demonstrated, surgical treatment is indicated. About one-third of
the angiograms are negative and probably indicate that thrombosis has taken
place in a small aneurysm. In such cases the treatment is conservative and the
prognosis good.

(See Chapter 12, *Lecture Notes on General Surgery*.)

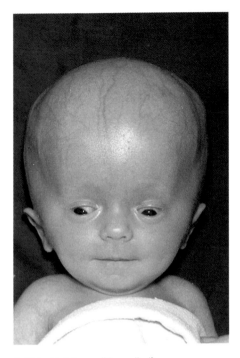

1 What is this condition called?
2 What is typical about the eyes?
3 Is papilloedema present in these children?
4 What other congenital abnormality is commonly associated with this?
5 What surgical procedure is used in its treatment?

1 Congenital hydrocephalus.

2 The eyeballs are displaced downwards. There may also be an associated squint and nystagmus.

3 No.

4 Spina bifida.

5 A ventriculo-atrial shunt using a Spitz–Holter valve.

(See Chapter 12, *Lecture Notes on General Surgery*.)

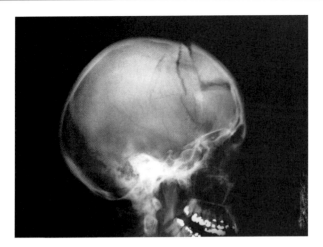

This is the lateral skull X-ray of a young man who came off his motorcycle and struck his forehead against the pavement.

1 What abnormality does the X-ray demonstrate?

2 This was a closed fracture; what sort of skull fracture is nearly always compound in the adult patient?

3 What type of skull fracture only occurs in children?

4 What discharge may the patient develop if the fracture involves the frontal or ethmoid sinuses, and what is the danger of this?

5 How is this discharge differentiated from nasal secretion?

1 A severe frontal fracture.

2 Depressed fractures in the adult are nearly always compound.

3 A 'pond' fracture.

4 Leakage of CSF from the nose (CSF rhinorrhoea). The danger of this is that the tear in the dura allows a pathway for infection via the nasal cavity to the meninges — meningitis.

5 The fluid is collected and tested for sugar. CSF contains sugar and no mucus, unlike nasal discharge, which contains little sugar and is rich in mucus. Jugular compression may increase the flow of CSF from the nose.

(See Chapter 13, *Lecture Notes on General Surgery*.)

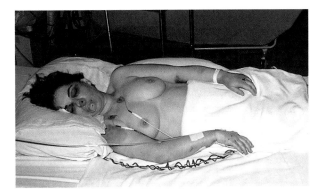

This patient was a pedestrian who was knocked down by a bus and admitted to hospital in deep coma.

1 What is the most important single thing to ensure on her admission to hospital?

2 How has this been achieved in her case?

3 In what position should she have been transported to hospital?

4 What is the simplest way of giving this unconscious patient food and drink?

5 What eye signs would indicate increasing intracranial compression?

1 The most important single factor in the care of the deeply unconscious patient, from whatever cause, is maintenance of the airway.

2 Nasal and oral airways are in place. This was sufficient to maintain adequate respiration and an endotracheal tube was not necessary.

3 The patient should be transported in the 'tonsil position' — placed on one side with the body tilted head downwards. This allows the tongue to fall forward and bronchial secretions, vomit or blood to drain from the mouth rather than be inhaled.

4 A fine naso-gastric tube is passed, which allows adequate hydration and nourishment, even in prolonged periods of unconsciousness.

5 Dilatation of the pupil and failure of its response to light on the side of cerebral compression. As compression continues, the opposite pupil in turn dilates and becomes fixed to light.

(See Chapter 13, *Lecture Notes on General Surgery*.)

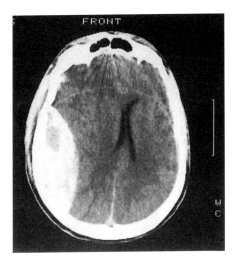

This is the CT scan of the skull of a young cricketer. He was hit on the head by a cricket ball, was knocked out, regained consciousness and then relapsed into coma 5 hours later.

1 What can you see on the CT scan?

2 What is the period of regained consciousness called?

3 What physical signs might have been found when the patient relapsed into coma?

4 Should a lumbar puncture be performed at this stage?

5 What urgent treatment is required here?

1 A localized collection of fluid is seen beneath the parietal bone — an extradural haematoma.

2 The 'lucid interval'.

3 A rising blood pressure, slowing pulse, dilatation of the pupil on the affected side, possibly hemiparesis or hemiplegia on the contralateral side. There may be a scalp haematoma over the site of the extradural clot.

4 No, this may produce 'coning' of the brain stem through the foramen magnum.

5 Maintain the airway, rapid transfer to theatre for craniotomy with evacuation of the clot and control of the bleeding meningeal vessel.

(See Chapter 13, *Lecture Notes on General Surgery*.)

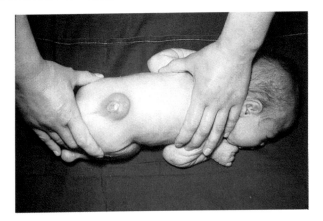

An obvious congenital lesion was found in this newborn baby.

1 What is it called?

2 What methods of antenatal screening are available for its detection?

3 What determines the prognosis of such cases?

4 What other congenital abnormality may typically co-exist with this?

5 What is its treatment?

1 Spina bifida with meningocele (protrusion of the meninges through the vertebral defect without nervous tissue involvement).

2 Alpha-feto protein level raised in amniotic fluid; ultrasound.

3 Whether neural tissue (cord or spinal roots) is involved—a myelomeningocele. This is often complicated by paraplegia and loss of sphincter control.

4 Hydrocephalus (see Fig. 31) nearly always co-exists with a myelomeningocele (the Arnold–Chiari malformation).

5 Surgical repair.

(See Chapter 14, *Lecture Notes on General Surgery*.)

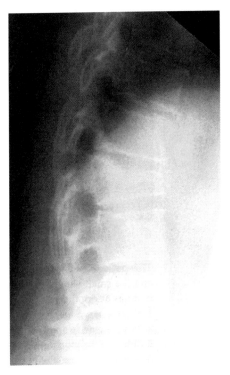

This is the lateral X-ray of the spine taken in casualty of a man, aged 40, who fell off some scaffolding at work, landing on his feet. He complained of severe dorsolumbar back pain. Fortunately, there was no evidence of any obvious neurological injury on clinical examination.

1 What fracture does the X-ray demonstrate?

2 What physical signs would you expect to find on examining the spine?

3 What type of fracture of the spine is likely to produce a spinal cord or spinal root injury?

4 Why is the incidence of spinal cord injury higher in cervical rather than in dorsolumbar fractures?

5 How would you treat this particular patient?

1 A wedge fracture of the body of the 12th thoracic vertebra.

2 Localized bruising, tenderness and often a kyphus at the site of the fracture.

3 An unstable fracture dislocation with forward or lateral displacement of the spine.

4 There is a much closer fit of the cervical cord within the vertebral canal compared with the wider lumbar region.

5 The patient is kept in bed for 2–3 weeks to allow the associated soft tissue injury to subside. This is followed by early exercise and active mobilization.

(See Chapter 14, *Lecture Notes on General Surgery*.)

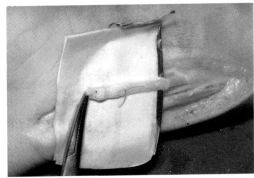

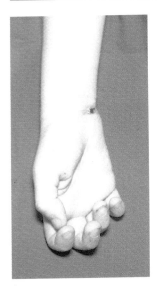

A

B

This patient's wrist was injured by a piece of broken glass and the small wound is clearly visible (A); (B) shows the findings at operation.

1 Which nerve has been injured?

2 What name is applied to this deformity?

3 What is the mechanism of this deformity?

4 What is the associated sensory loss?

5 Describe a reliable clinical test for the muscle weakness.

I The ulnar nerve.

2 Clawed hand or *main en griffe*.

3 The clawed appearance results from the unopposed action of the long flexors and extensors of the fingers. This results from paralysis of all the intrinsic muscles of the hand apart from the muscles of the thenar eminence and the two lateral lumbricals, which are supplied by the median nerve.

4 The ulnar border of the hand and ulnar one and a half fingers.

5 The patient is unable to abduct and adduct the fingers of the hand laid flat, palm downwards, on the table. In particular, he is unable to grip a piece of paper placed between the fingers.

(See Chapter 15, *Lecture Notes on General Surgery*.)

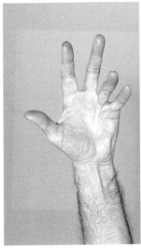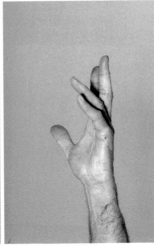

This is a common deformity, particularly in elderly men, although it is sometimes found in women.

1 What is it called? Correct spelling please!
2 What is responsible for this deformity?
3 Which fingers are usually affected?
4 Which part of the finger escapes?
5 Is it associated with any other contracture?

1 Dupuytren's contracture.

2 Fibrosis of the palmar aponeurosis.

3 This usually starts at the ring finger, spreads to the fifth finger and sometimes to the middle finger. Only rarely are the index finger or thumb implicated.

4 Since the aponeurosis only extends to the base of the middle phalanx, the distal interphalangeal joint escapes.

5 About 10% of patients have an associated contracture of the plantar fascia.

(See Chapter 15, *Lecture Notes on General Surgery*.)

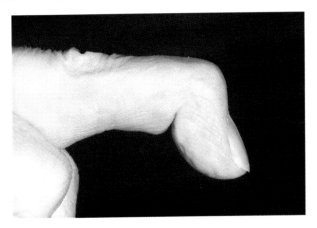

This young man has a characteristic deformity of his right index finger.

1 What is it called?
2 What causes it?
3 What is the sport which is classically associated with this?
4 How may it be treated?

1 Mallet finger.

2 Avulsion of the extensor tendon at its insertion with the base of the distal phalanx (or a flake fracture of the base of the phalanx).

3 Cricketer.

4 Immobilize the finger with the distal interphalangeal joint extended in a mallet finger splint. If there is a fracture of the distal phalanx, this may be fixed by means of a pin.

(See Chapter 15, *Lecture Notes on General Surgery*.)

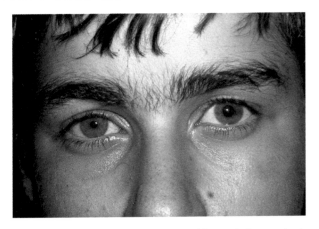

This young man of 17 years underwent a right cervical sympathectomy.

1 What is the name of the abnormality affecting his right eye?

2 What is the anatomical structure which, when damaged, produces this syndrome?

3 What causes the pupillary abnormality?

4 What causes the eyelid abnormality?

5 How may the skin on the right side of the face be affected?

1 Horner's syndrome.

2 Damage to the first thoracic segment contribution to the cervical sympathetic chain.

3 The pupil is constricted due to paralysis of the dilator pupillae, which receives sympathetic innervation.

4 The ptosis is due to paralysis of the sympathetic fibres supplying levator palpebrae superioris via the oculomotor nerve.

5 Loss of sweating (under sympathetic control).

(See Chapter 15, *Lecture Notes on General Surgery*.)

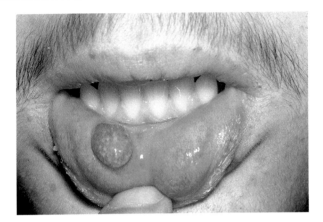

This young man presented with a painless, blue cystic lesion on his lip.

1 What is this called?

2 What is its aetiology?

3 These cysts contain clear colourless mucus — why then do they appear blue?

4 How does the cyst usually bother the patient?

5 What treatment would you advise?

1 Mucous retention cyst of the lip.

2 Leakage of mucus submucosally due to minor trauma to the mucous glands of the lip.

3 Reflected light — in the same way that the sea appears to be green or blue.

4 It tends to get bitten.

5 Surgical excision.

(See Chapter 16, *Lecture Notes on General Surgery*.)

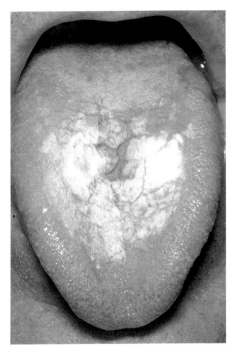

1   What is the name given to this lesion of the tongue?
2   Where else may this condition occur?
3   What mnemonic covers its aetiological factors?
4   What is the importance of this condition?
5   How should it be treated?

1 Leukoplakia (literally, a white plaque).

2 Anywhere within the mouth, but other sites where it may be found are the larynx, the anus and the vulva.

3 Although often no cause can be found, remember the list of S's: syphilis, smoking, sepsis, sore tooth, spirits and spices. These are also predisposing factors to cancers within the mouth.

4 It is often premalignant — suspect this if there is local thickening, pain, bleeding or areas of erythema.

5 Remove any underlying cause. Biopsy any suspicious area for malignant change. Surgical or diathermy excision.

(See Chapter 16, *Lecture Notes on General Surgery*.)

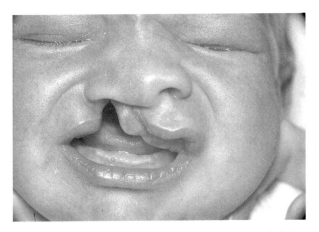

This photograph shows two obvious and common congenital abnormalities.

1 What are they called?

2 How often do they co-exist?

3 Why is it important to carry out a careful general examination of this child?

4 What is the immediate problem presented by the palatal defect?

5 How should this child be treated?

1 Cleft lip and palate.

2 In roughly 50% of cases; 25% have a cleft lip alone, 25% a cleft palate alone.

3 10% have other congenital anomalies.

4 Interference with normal sucking. The infant requires careful spoon or bottle feeding by a skilled nurse.

5 Early surgical repair; first the lip and then the palate.

(See Chapter 16, *Lecture Notes on General Surgery*.)

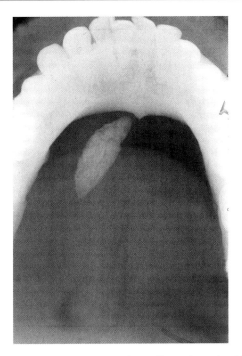

This patient complained of a swelling at the angle of the jaw, which enlarged and became painful after meals.

1 What does this X-ray demonstrate?
2 Does this occur in other salivary glands?
3 What is the chemical composition of this lesion?
4 How would you palpate this?
5 Is anything known about its aetiology?

1 A calculus in the duct of the submandibular salivary gland.

2 Rarely in the parotid, never in the sublingual gland.

3 Calcium phosphate and carbonate. The high calcium content means that these stones are nearly always radio-opaque.

4 By bimanual palpation—the index finger of one hand in the floor of the mouth, the index finger of the other beneath the angle of the jaw.

5 Not really. These calculi are nearly always associated with a clean and well kept mouth; a possible explanation is that the calculi develop around minute fragments of toothpaste.

(See Chapter 16, *Lecture Notes on General Surgery*.)

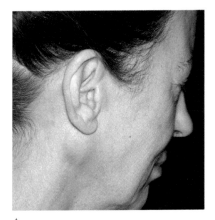

A

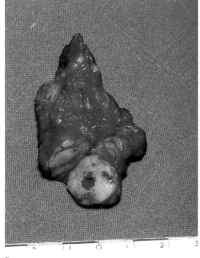

B

This patient presented with a very slowly enlarging, painless lump just below the external auditory meatus. Clinically it lay within the parotid gland (A). A photograph of the surgically excised specimen is shown in (B).

1 What is the likely diagnosis?

2 Having examined the lump itself, what other procedures must you perform in the clinical examination of a parotid swelling?

3 Does this tumour affect other salivary glands?

4 What does it look like under the microscope?

5 Although the tumour is apparently encapsulated, why has it been removed with a cuff of surrounding gland?

1 Pleomorphic adenoma of the parotid.

2 (a) Inspect the parotid duct.

(b) Test the facial nerve.

(c) Inspect and palpate the fauces—a parotid tumour may plunge into the pharynx.

(d) Palpate the regional lymph nodes.

3 90% of these tumours occur in the parotid, but they may occasionally be found in the submandibular or sublingual glands, or in the accessory salivary glands scattered over the inside of the mouth.

4 Glandular acini within a blue-staining stroma.

5 The apparent capsule is often breached by 'amoeboid' processes, which may be left behind if simple enucleation is performed; recurrence would then be inevitable.

(See Chapter 17, *Lecture Notes on General Surgery*.)

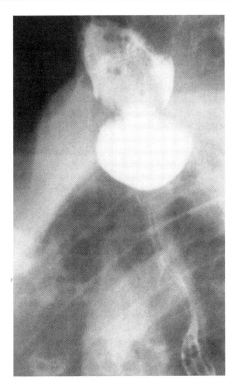

This is the barium swallow of a patient in his 60s who complained of several years of progressive difficulty in swallowing. He found that food tended to stick in his throat and he regurgitated food he had recently swallowed.

I What condition does the X-ray demonstrate?

2 Where is the pouch situated anatomically?

3 What is its presumed aetiology?

4 As it enlarges, what does the pouch do to the oesophagus, and why is this important?

5 How is this condition treated surgically?

1 Pharyngeal pouch.

2 It is a mucosal protrusion between the two parts of the inferior pharyngeal constrictor—the thyropharyngeus and the cricopharyngeus (Killian's dehiscence).

3 It is believed to result from spasm of cricopharyngeus.

4 As the pouch enlarges, it displaces the oesophagus laterally. This means that an oesophageal catheter, an oesophagoscope or a bougie will tend to enter the pouch rather than pass down the oesophagus itself; the pouch may thus be perforated.

5 Surgical excision of the pouch combined with myotomy of the cricopharyngeus muscle.

(See Chapter 18, *Lecture Notes on General Surgery*.)

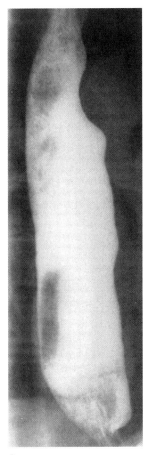

A

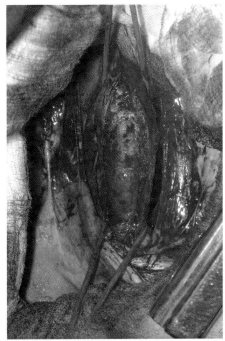

B

A 45-year-old woman presented with a history of slowly progressive dysphagia over the past few years. (A) demonstrates her barium swallow X-ray and (B) is a photograph taken at left thoracotomy after the operative procedure had been completed.

I Describe what the barium swallow shows.

2 What is this disease called?

3 What is its cause?

4 What may a plain X-ray of the chest show in an advanced stage of this condition?

5 What operative procedure has been performed in (B)?

1 There is gross dilatation and tortuosity of the oesophagus leading to a narrowed segment at its lower end. As well as barium, the oesophagus contains a good deal of food debris.

2 Achalasia of the cardia.

3 There is a neuromuscular failure of relaxation at the lower end of the oesophagus with incoordination of peristalsis of the oesophagus above, which leads to progressive oesophageal dilatation and tortuosity.

4 The dilated oesophagus may produce the appearance of a mediastinal mass and there may be evidence of pneumonitis from aspiration of gastric contents.

5 A Heller's operation (cardiomyotomy). The muscle of the lower end of the oesophagus has been split longitudinally down to the mucosa.

(See Chapter 18, *Lecture Notes on General Surgery*.)

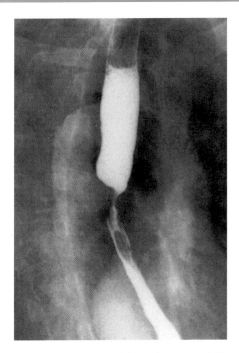

This is a barium swallow X-ray of a man aged 65 years.

1 What lesion does it demonstrate?

2 How can the diagnosis be confirmed?

3 What would be the histology of this lesion?

4 What would be the most likely presenting feature that brought this patient to his doctor?

5 Where would you palpate to detect possibly involved lymph nodes?

 1 A carcinoma of the middle one-third of the oesophagus.
 2 Oesophagoscopy with biopsy.
 3 A squamous carcinoma.
 4 Dysphagia of recent origin.
 5 The supraclavicular fossae — particularly the left (Troissier's sign).

(See Chapter 18, *Lecture Notes on General Surgery*.)

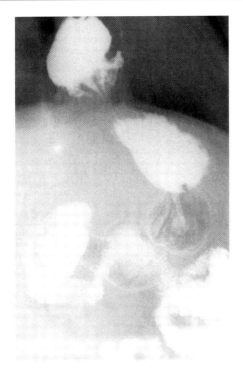

This is a barium meal performed on a woman aged 50 years.

1 What condition does this demonstrate?
2 In what position is the patient?
3 What produces this appearance?
4 In what sort of person is this condition particularly common?
5 What symptoms may be associated with it?

1 A sliding hiatus hernia.

2 The patient is tipped head down on the X-ray table.

3 In this position the stomach slides through the hiatus of the diaphragm into the chest. Note that the fundus of the stomach is filled with barium.

4 An obese, middle-aged or elderly woman.

5 The condition is often entirely symptomless. Associated reflux produces a burning retrosternal or epigastric pain, which is aggravated by lying down or stooping. Long-standing oesophagitis may result in stricture formation and bleeding. A very large hernia may produce mechanical effects—particularly cough and breathlessness.

(See Chapter 19, *Lecture Notes on General Surgery*.)

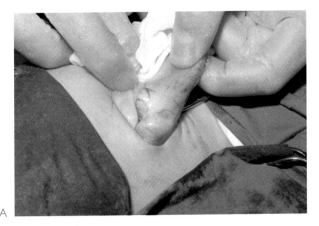

A

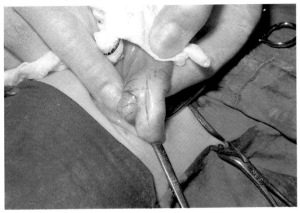

B

These photographs were taken at operation on the pylorus of a baby boy aged
3 weeks.

1 What pathological condition of the pylorus is shown in (A)?

2 What would be the typical symptoms in such a case?

3 What might you have found in your pre-operative clinical examination of this
baby?

4 What is the name of the operation being performed in (B), and what does
this comprise?

5 What is the prognosis in such a case?

1 Congenital hypertrophic pyloric stenosis.

2 The baby is usually male (80%), first born (50%) and the condition often occurs in siblings. The baby is usually between the ages of 3 and 4 weeks, although symptoms may present rarely at, or soon after birth. The principal symptom is projectile vomiting. There is failure to gain weight and the baby is constipated.

3 There may be obvious dehydration. Visible peristalsis in the dilated stomach may be seen in the epigastrium. A palpable pyloric tumour may be felt in the right upper abdomen (especially after vomiting a feed) in 95% of cases.

4 Ramstedt's operation. A longitudinal incision is made through the hypertrophied pyloric muscle down to the mucosa.

5 The mortality should be zero and the long-term results are excellent.

(See Chapter 20, *Lecture Notes on General Surgery*.)

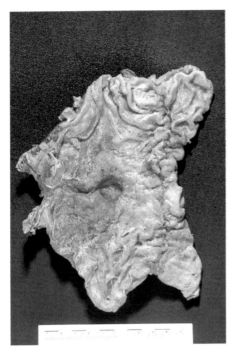

This is a specimen of a stomach resected at partial gastrectomy and laid open.

1 What is the naked-eye diagnosis here?

2 What features suggest that the ulcer is benign?

3 What are the typical symptoms you would expect this patient to have experienced?

4 What complications may result from this lesion?

5 What would be the indications for advising surgery in a patient with this disease?

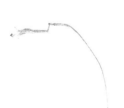

1 A probably benign gastric ulcer.

2 The site is typical for a benign ulcer—approximately mid-lesser curve—and there is no thickening or heaping up the edges of the ulcer to suggest a carcinoma.

3 Episodes of epigastric pain interspersed with periods of relief. Pain coming on after food or preceding a meal, characteristically waking the patient in the early hours of the morning and relieved by milk and antacids.

4 (a) Perforation—either into the general peritoneal cavity or into adjacent structures, e.g. pancreas, liver or colon.

(b) Stenosis.

(c) Haemorrhage.

(d) Malignant change.

5 Failure to respond to medical treatment, perforation, haemorrhage or malignant change.

(See Chapter 20, *Lecture Notes on General Surgery*.)

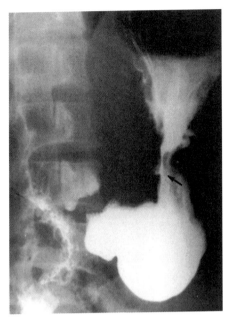

This is the barium meal of a 60-year-old woman. The lesion on the lesser curve, indicated by an arrow, was constant on all the films.

1 What do you see here?

2 What other condition must be considered in the differential diagnosis of this appearance?

3 What investigation needs to be performed to confirm the diagnosis?

4 What is the incidence of this lesion compared with duodenal ulcers?

1 A niche on the otherwise quite smooth line of the lesser curvature of the stomach — this has the appearance of a benign gastric ulcer.

2 A carcinoma of the stomach.

3 Gastroscopy with biopsy in order to differentiate between a benign ulcer and a carcinoma of the stomach.

4 Duodenal ulcer is much commoner.

(See Chapter 20, *Lecture Notes on General Surgery.*)

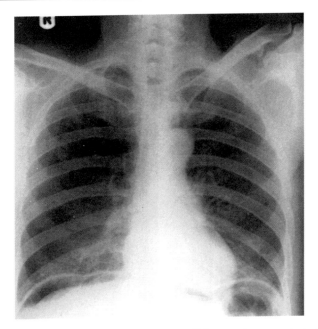

This is the chest X-ray of a young man of 30 years who presented with sudden onset of extremely severe generalized abdominal pain.

1 What does the X-ray demonstrate?
2 What is the most likely cause of this?
3 Is this X-ray appearance invariably present in this emergency?
4 This patient complained of pain over the right shoulder — why?
5 How is the patient to be treated?

1 Free gas below the diaphragm.

2 In a young man of this age and with this story, a perforated peptic ulcer—most probably a duodenal ulcer.

3 No, free gas is only present in about 70% of cases of perforated peptic ulcer.

4 Referred pain via the phrenic nerve from subdiaphragmatic irritation.

5 The patient is reassured, opiate analgesia is given, an intravenous drip commenced, antibiotic therapy initiated and surgical repair of the perforation performed.

(See Chapter 20, *Lecture Notes on General Surgery*.)

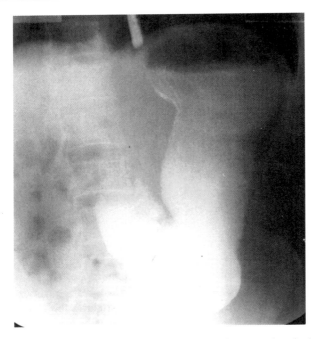

This is the barium meal of a man, aged 53, who is known to have had a duodenal ulcer for many years.

1 What gross abnormality does it demonstrate?
2 What would be the likely presenting symptoms of this?
3 What physical signs might you elicit on examining this patient's abdomen?
4 What metabolic disturbances may occur in this condition?
5 How would these metabolic disturbances be corrected?

1 Pyloric stenosis. The stomach is enormously enlarged and contains a considerable quantity of gastric residue.

2 Profuse vomiting. The vomitus may contain food eaten 1 or 2 days previously. There is associated loss of weight. There may be constipation because of dehydration and there may be weakness due to electrolyte disturbance.

3 A gastric splash, visible gastric peristalsis and, in gross cases such as this, a hypertrophied stomach full of stale food and fluid can be palpated.

4 Dehydration. Serum chloride, sodium and potassium may be lowered and plasma bicarbonate and urea raised. Urine is concentrated, initially alkaline, later acid; its chloride content is reduced or absent.

5 Intravenous replacement with saline and added potassium.

(See Chapter 20, *Lecture Notes on General Surgery*.)

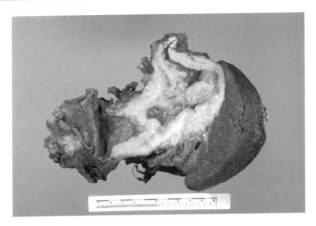

This is the specimen obtained by a total gastrectomy and splenectomy.

1 What are the names (one English, one Latin) given to this form of gastric carcinoma?

2 What produces this characteristic appearance?

3 How common is carcinoma of the stomach in the United Kingdom and what is happening to its incidence?

4 Is anything known about the aetiology of gastric carcinoma?

5 What is the prognosis of gastric carcinoma, and on what factors does this depend?

1 Leather bottle stomach or linitis plastica.

2 This appearance is caused by submucous infiltration of the tumour with marked fibrous reaction. This produces a small, thickened, contracted stomach without, or with only superficial, ulceration.

3 Gastric carcinoma is the fifth commonest cause of deaths from cancer in the United Kingdom but, for unknown reasons, its incidence is decreasing.

4 There is a definite link with subjects having blood group A, the incidence is raised in patients with pernicious anaemia, and occasionally a gastric carcinoma arises in a previous chronic gastric ulcer. There is no absolute association with diet, alcohol or tobacco. The disease is particularly common in the Japanese. However, nothing is really understood about its aetiology.

5 Prognosis depends on the extent of spread and the degree of anaplasia of the tumour, together with the general fitness of the patient for surgery. Overall prognosis is poor, with only 5% of all cases surviving for 5 years. However, those who undergo 'curative' surgery have a 20% 5-year survival.

(See Chapter 20, *Lecture Notes on General Surgery*.)

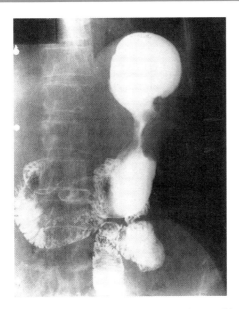

This is the barium meal of a middle-aged man with a recent history of epigastric discomfort and loss of weight. The X-ray appearances seen here were constant on all the films taken.

1 Describe what the X-ray demonstrates.
2 What is the probable diagnosis?
3 What investigation is now needed to confirm this diagnosis?
4 What clinical evidence may be found of lymphatic spread of this tumour?
5 What abdominal signs would you look for that would indicate:
   (a) Portal vein spread.
   (b) Transcoelomic spread?

1 There is a constant narrowing of the body of the stomach.
2 Carcinoma of the stomach.
3 Fibreoptic gastroscopy with biopsy.
4 Enlarged hard left supraclavicular lymph nodes of Virchow (Troissier's sign).
5 (a) Enlargement of the liver, with or without jaundice, together with ascites.
   (b) Ascites.

(See Chapter 20, *Lecture Notes on General Surgery*.)

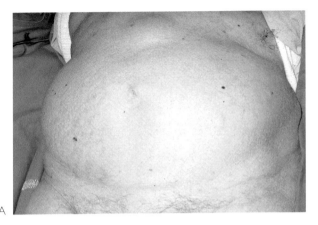

A

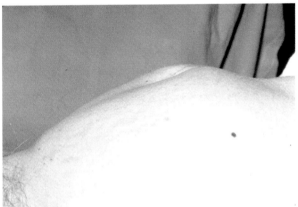

B

This is the appearance of the abdomen of an 80-year-old woman, who presented with a 48-hour history of central colicky abdominal pain and absolute constipation. The abdomen, as you can see, is considerably distended. In the last few hours she has commenced to vomit copiously.

1 What is your clinical diagnosis?
2 What special investigation could you order to help confirm your diagnosis?
3 Name three common causes of this emergency in elderly patients.
4 What is meant by *absolute* constipation?
5 What pre-operative treatment would you institute in this patient?

1 Acute intestinal obstruction.

2 Plain X-rays of the abdomen (erect and supine) are helpful in confirming the diagnosis and localizing the site of the obstruction (see Figs A and B, Question 58). It is important to note, however, that a small percentage of patients with intestinal obstruction show no abnormality on plain X-rays of the abdomen.

3 Strangulated inguinal or femoral hernia, carcinoma of the large bowel, diverticular disease of the colon.

4 Failure to pass flatus in addition to stool.

5 (a) Reassure the patient.

(b) Relieve pain with morphine or pethidine pre-medication.

(c) Nasogastric suction.

(d) Intravenous replacement of fluid and electrolytes.

(e) Commence prophylactic antibiotic therapy.

(See Chapter 21, *Lecture Notes on General Surgery*.)

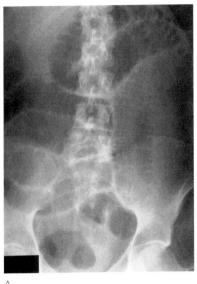

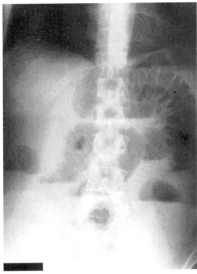

A

B

This patient had undergone an appendicectomy 2 years previously. He was then admitted with acute abdominal pain and distension. These are his plain abdominal X-rays.

1 In what position was the patient X-rayed in (A) and in (B)?

2 What does the X-ray in (A) demonstrate?

3 What accounts for the appearances in X-ray (B)?

4 How do you distinguish radiologically between distended small and large intestine?

5 From the history given, what is the probable cause of this emergency?

1 X-ray (A) is in the supine position and X-ray (B) is taken with the patient erect.

2 Distended loops of small intestine.

3 With the patient in the erect position, gas in the distended loops of the small intestine rises to the top of the contained fluid, thus producing this appearance of multiple fluid levels.

4 Small bowel is suggested by a ladder pattern of dilated loops which take up a central position in the abdomen and by striations which pass completely across the width of the distended loop as a result of the circular mucosal folds in the small intestine. Distended large bowel tends to lie peripherally and to show the haustrations of the taenia coli, which do not extend across the whole width of the bowel.

5 Small bowel obstruction in the presence of evidence of a previous operation immediately suggests adhesions as the cause.

(See Chapter 21, *Lecture Notes on General Surgery*.)

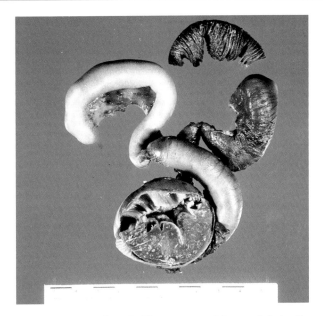

This is a segment of terminal ileum removed from an infant with neonatal intestinal obstruction.

1 What is the cause of the obstruction?
2 What is the underlying pathology which results in this condition?
3 What are the typical X-ray appearances of the abdomen in these cases?
4 What may happen to the obstructed segment of bowel?
5 How may the obstruction be treated?

I Meconium ileus.

2 This is a neonatal manifestation of 10–15% of infants with cystic fibrosis. Because of the loss of intestinal mucus and a blockage of pancreatic ducts with consequent loss of tryptic digestion, the lower ileum of the fetus becomes blocked with inspissated sticky meconium.

3 Distended coils of small intestine with the typical mottled 'ground glass' appearance of meconium.

4 Perforation of the bowel may occur in intra-uterine life (meconium peritonitis). The impacted segment of ileum may develop areas of gangrene from pressure necrosis.

5 It may be possible to clear the meconium by instillation of Gastrograffin per rectum under X-ray control. If this fails, or if the bowel has perforated, surgery is required. It may be possible to open the bowel and remove the inspissated meconium by lavage, but occasionally the impacted segment may show areas of gangrene and requires resection, as in this case.

(See Chapter 22, *Lecture Notes on General Surgery.*)

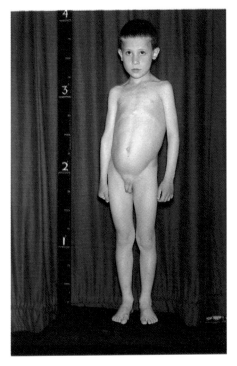

This boy is actually 15 years old, although he appears much younger. He presented with a life-long history of stubborn constipation.

1 What do you notice about the abdomen?

2 What is the diagnosis? Give both the eponym and the scientific name.

3 What is the pathological basis of this condition and how is this demonstrated in practice?

4 What is the sex distribution of this disease?

5 What is its surgical management?

I The abdomen is grossly distended.

2 Hirschsprung's disease or congenital megacolon.

3 There is faulty development of the parasympathetic innervation of the distal bowel. There is an absence of ganglion cells in the plexuses of Auerbach and Meissner in the rectum. This deficiency sometimes extends into the lower colon and rarely affects the whole of the large bowel. The involved segment is spastic with gross proximal distension of the colon. A biopsy of the rectal wall shows complete absence of ganglion cells and is diagnostic.

4 80% of the patients are male.

5 If the child is obstructed in the neonatal period a colostomy is performed. Definitive surgery comprises resection of the aganglionic segment with a pull-through anastomosis performed between the normal colon above and the anal canal below.

(See Chapter 22, *Lecture Notes on General Surgery.*)

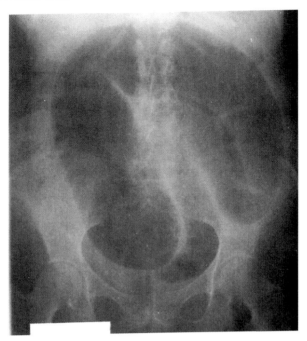

An elderly patient presented with acute intestinal obstruction. On examination his abdomen was grossly distended.

1 Describe what you see in this X-ray of the patient's abdomen.

2 What is the diagnosis?

3 This emergency is relatively unusual in the United Kingdom. In which parts of the world is it much commoner?

4 What other hollow organs may undergo this process?

5 Left untreated, what would happen to this patient?

1 There is an enormously dilated oval gas shadow looped on itself to give the typical 'bent inner-tube' sign.

2 Volvulus of the sigmoid colon.

3 Volvulus of the sigmoid is much commoner in Russia, Scandinavia and Central Africa than in the United Kingdom.

4 Volvulus may also affect the caecum, small intestine, gall bladder and stomach.

5 Untreated, the strangulated bowel undergoes gangrene, leading to death from peritonitis.

(See Chapter 22, *Lecture Notes on General Surgery*.)

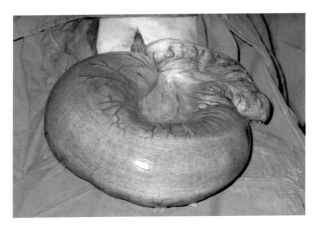

This is the operative finding in the patient whose X-ray is shown in Question 61.

1 Describe the pathology that is being demonstrated.

2 What conservative method was employed (unsuccessfully, it so happens) to try to avoid emergency surgery?

3 What sort of patient is likely to suffer this emergency?

4 What are the factors that may precipitate a volvulus of the intestine?

5 What must be done to prevent the volvulus from recurring?

1 There is an enormously distended sigmoid loop, which has undergone volvulus.

2 A rectal tube was passed through the sigmoidoscope. This often untwists an early volvulus, with passage of vast amounts of flatus.

3 The patient is usually elderly and constipated. Men are affected four times more commonly than women.

4 Precipitating factors for volvulus of the intestine include:

    (a) An abnormally mobile loop of intestine.

    (b) An abnormally loaded loop (e.g. the sigmoid colon in chronic constipation).

    (c) A loop fixed at its apex by adhesions.

    (d) A loop of bowel with a narrow base.

5 Elective resection of the redundant sigmoid loop should be performed to prevent recurrent volvulus.

(See Chapter 22, *Lecture Notes on General Surgery*.)

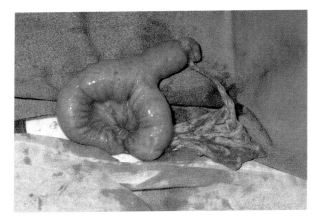

This diverticulum of the small intestine was found at laparotomy.

1 What is it called?

2 What is its embryological origin?

3 Where is it found in the small intestine, and how common is it?

4 Name the ways in which it may present clinically.

5 How may it cause a child to pass melaena stools?

1 Meckel's diverticulum.

2 It is the remnant of the vitello-intestinal duct.

3 It lies on the antemesenteric border of the ileum, about 0.6 m (2 feet) from the ileocaecal valve, and occurs in about 2% of the population.

4 It may present in numerous ways:

(a) A symptomless finding at operation or autopsy.

(b) Acute inflammation.

(c) Perforation by a foreign body.

(d) Intussusception.

(e) Peptic ulceration with haemorrhage or perforation.

(f) An umbilical fistula.

(g) Raspberry tumour at the umbilicus.

(h) A vitello-intestinal band from the tip of the Meckel to the umbilicus may snare a loop of intestine to produce obstruction or act as the apex of a volvulus.

5 The diverticulum may contain heterotopic gastric epithelium secreting hydrochloric acid. This produces a peptic ulcer and characteristically is the cause of melaena about the age of 10 years.

(See Chapter 23, *Lecture Notes on General Surgery*.)

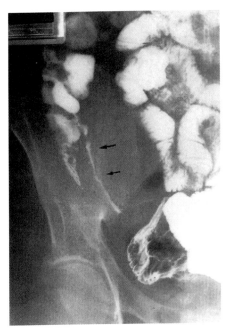

This is the barium meal and follow-through X-ray examination of a young man of 28, who presented with right iliac fossa pain and diarrhoea. Examination revealed a tender mass in the right iliac fossa.

1 What is the name given to the long strictured segment of terminal ileum (arrowed)?

2 What disease characteristically produces this appearance?

3 What other radiological features may be seen in the affected segment of bowel?

4 What other parts of the alimentary tract may be affected by this condition?

5 Is anything definitely known about its aetiology?

1 The string sign of Kantor.

2 Crohn's disease.

3 Fine ulceration may be seen, giving the so-called 'rose-thorn' appearance of the mucosa.

4 Any part of the alimentary tract from the mouth to the anus may be affected by Crohn's disease.

5 The aetiology is unknown, although acute regional ileitis can be caused by the bacterium *Yersinia enterocolitica*.

(See Chapter 23, *Lecture Notes on General Surgery*.)

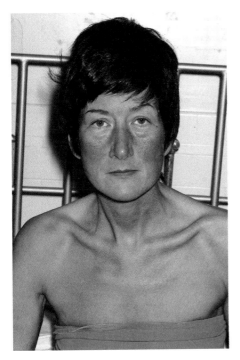

This woman had a tumour resected from her terminal ileum 5 years previously. At that time, the regional lymph nodes were involved. This time she presented with a grossly enlarged liver and with this extraordinary appearance.

1 What is the name of this syndrome?
2 What is the commonest site of the primary tumour?
3 What other features may be present in this condition?
4 What special investigation is performed to confirm the diagnosis?
5 How may the liver secondaries be treated in such a case?

1 The carcinoid syndrome.

2 The appendix is the commonest site of carcinoid, although here the tumour is relatively benign and only 4% eventually metastasize.

3 As well as the enlarged liver and the flushing with attacks of cyanosis, there may be diarrhoea with noisy borborygmi, bronchospasm and pulmonary stenosis.

4 5-hydroxytryptamine is excreted in the urine as 5-hydroxyindole acetic acid (5-HIAA). This can be estimated by paper chromatography.

5 It may be possible to resect the liver secondaries. More extensive deposits can be treated by embolization of the hepatic arterial supply. Cytotoxic therapy may induce worthwhile remission. Symptoms may be controlled using 5HT antagonists, e.g. methysergide.

(See Chapter 23, *Lecture Notes on General Surgery.*)

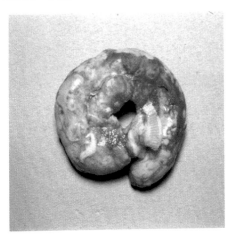

This specimen shows a gangrenous perforated appendix removed at operation.

1 Are there any specific laboratory tests that confirm the clinical diagnosis of acute appendicitis?

2 Does the presence of pus cells in the urine exclude this diagnosis?

3 If perforation occurs, must the patient inevitably develop a generalized peritonitis?

4 What physical signs would suggest a general peritonitis?

5 How is peritonitis due to a perforated appendix managed?

1 No; there is usually a polymorph leucocytosis, but this is neither specific nor invariable.

2 Although pus cells in the urine would suggest a urinary tract infection, an inflamed appendix adherent to the ureter or bladder may produce microscopic haematuria or pyuria.

3 No; the appendix may be walled-off into an appendix mass.

4 The temperature and pulse are raised, the patient is flushed and toxic, the tongue is coated, the abdomen is diffusely tender and rigid with absent bowel sounds.

5 Appendicectomy, supplemented by nasogastric aspiration, intravenous fluid replacement and antibiotic therapy.

(See Chapter 24, *Lecture Notes on General Surgery.*)

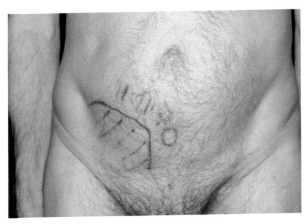

This patient, a previously healthy man of 23 years, presented with a 5-day history of acute pain in the lower right abdomen. The mass which was felt has been outlined.

1 What is the most likely diagnosis?

2 What features in the history might suggest that this mass was due to Crohn's disease involving the terminal ileum?

3 What other common disease would be considered in the differential diagnosis if this patient was aged 73?

4 Describe the initial treatment of an appendix mass.

5 If the mass settles, what would you then advise?

1 An appendix mass.

2 Crohn's disease would be considered if there had been a previous history of diarrhoea, often with loss of weight.

3 Carcinoma of the caecum.

4 Initially conservative treatment. The outline of the mass is marked on the skin, the patient put on bed rest and on fluids. Metronidazole is commenced. A careful watch should be kept on his general condition, temperature and pulse. On this regime 80% of appendix masses resolve. In the remaining cases the abscess enlarges over the next day or two and the temperature fails to subside. In these circumstances, drainage of the abscess is necessary.

5 If resolution occurs, then appendicectomy is carried out after an interval of 2 or 3 months to allow the inflammatory condition to settle completely. This is to prevent the risk of a further attack of acute appendicitis.

(See Chapter 24, *Lecture Notes on General Surgery.*)

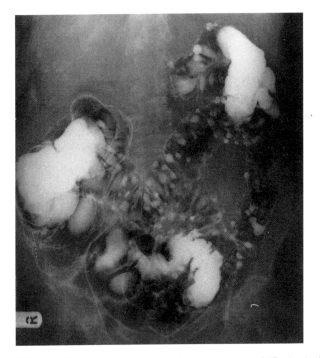

This is the barium enema of a symptomless woman of 65 who had this performed as part of a 'check up'.

1 What pathology does it show?
2 How common is this lesion in people of this age in the Western world?
3 Is there any known cause for this?
4 What are the common complications of this condition?
5 Is there any advice you would give this patient as a result of her X-ray?

1 Extensive diverticula of the colon.

2 About 30%.

3 The modern refined low roughage diet may be responsible for the thickening of the colon wall, which is the primary lesion in this condition.

4 An inflamed diverticulum may perforate into the general peritoneal cavity or may form a pericolic abscess. It may fistulate into adjacent structures (bladder, small bowel, vagina). Chronic infection and inflammatory fibrosis may result in obstructive symptoms, and there may be haemorrhage as a result of erosion of a vessel in the bowel wall.

5 A high roughage diet should be advised.

(See Chapter 25, *Lecture Notes on General Surgery.*)

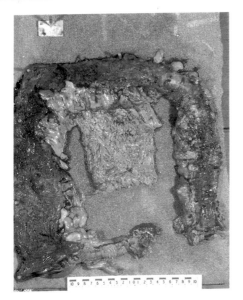

This is the colon removed from a young doctor of 25 with a long history of copious bloody diarrhoea.

1 What condition is shown?
2 What special investigations are performed to confirm the diagnosis?
3 What are the local complications of this condition?
4 What general complications may affect the patient?
5 What are the indications for total colectomy in this disease?

1 Ulcerative colitis—note that the whole length of the bowel is affected.

2 Sigmoidoscopy and biopsy, a barium enema examination and, if necessary, colonoscopy to inspect the whole of the large bowel.

3 Toxic dilatation, leading to perforation; haemorrhage; stricture formation; malignant change; perianal abscesses and fistula *in ano*.

4 Toxaemia; loss of weight; anaemia; arthritis; pyoderma; iritis and leg ulceration.

5 (a) Fulminating disease not responding to medical treatment.

   (b) Chronic disease not responding to medical treatment.

   (c) In long-standing disease as prophylactic against malignant change.

   (d) For the local and general complications listed above.

(See Chapter 25, *Lecture Notes on General Surgery.*)

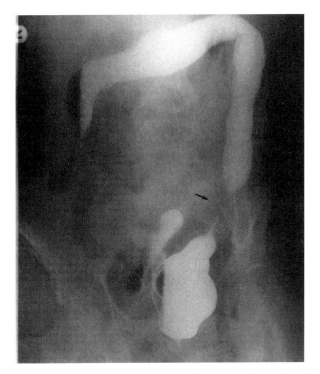

This is the barium enema of a man of 58 years. He has suffered episodes of bloody diarrhoea over the last 20 years and has now been admitted with a particularly severe episode. On examination a mass could be felt in his left lower abdomen (the appearances on this X-ray were constant throughout the whole series of films taken).

1 Describe your observations on this X-ray.

2 What is the underlying chronic disease here—and what complication has probably arisen from it, demonstrated by the arrow?

3 What further investigation will be necessary to confirm these two pathologies?

4 Which patients are particularly likely to develop the complication demonstrated here?

1 The whole of the colon has lost its normal haustrations and its lumen is narrowed throughout — the so-called 'drain pipe' colon. Fine ulceration can be seen along the ascending colon. There is a long stricture in the sigmoid colon.

2 Chronic ulcerative colitis with carcinomatous change in the sigmoid colon. Although non-malignant strictures may occur in ulcerative colitis, the fact that this patient has a mass in the left iliac fossa strongly suggests that this is a neoplastic stricture.

3 Colonoscopy with biopsy of the colonic mucosa and also of the strictured area. In this case, the biopsy material confirmed these two diagnoses.

4 The risk of malignant change in ulcerative colitis is greatest in long-standing and continuous colitis that affects the whole bowel, especially if symptoms commence in childhood or adolescence. It is estimated that 12% of patients with colitis of 20 years duration are likely to develop malignant change.

(See Chapter 25, *Lecture Notes on General Surgery.*)

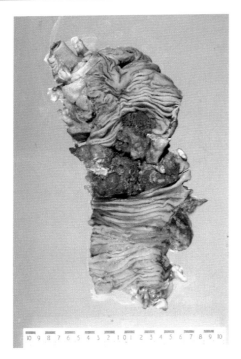

This specimen demonstrates the terminal ileum, caecum and ascending colon removed at right hemicolectomy.

1 Describe the macroscopic pathology that is demonstrated.

2 What is the microscopic nature of this tumour?

3 How do tumours in the right colon commonly present?

4 How do these symptoms differ from those that usually occur in carcinomas affecting the left side of the colon?

5 Describe the pathways of spread of this tumour.

1 There is a papilliferous tumour in the ascending colon.

2 An adenocarcinoma.

3 On the right side of the colon the stools are semi-liquid, the tumours tend to be proliferative and therefore obstructive symptoms are relatively uncommon. These patients often present with anaemia (due to chronic blood loss) and loss of weight.

4 Typically tumours of the left side of the colon are constricting growths and the contained stool is solid, therefore obstructive features predominate.

5 (a) *Local*: encircling the bowel wall and invading adjacent viscera.

(b) *Lymphatic*: to the regional lymph nodes with late involvement of the supraclavicular nodes via the thoracic duct.

(d) *Bloodstream*: spread to the liver via the portal vein, thence to the lungs.

(e) *Transcoelomic*: with deposits of nodules throughout the peritoneal cavity and with ascites.

(See Chapter 25, *Lecture Notes on General Surgery*.)

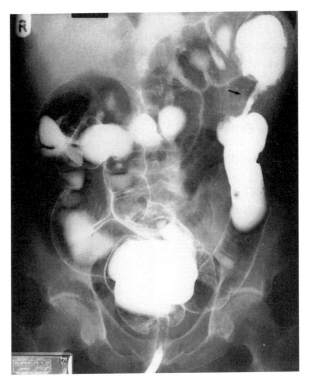

This is the barium enema of a man, aged 70, who presented with altered bowel habit and rectal bleeding.

1 What is the most likely pathology demonstrated here (arrowed)?
2 How can this lesion be visualized and a biopsy taken?
3 How common is this disease in the United Kingdom?
4 What are the predisposing factors which may lead to this condition?
5 What common emergency results from this lesion?

I Carcinoma of the descending colon.

2 Fibreoptic colonoscopy.

3 Carcinoma of the large bowel is the second commonest cause of deaths from cancer in the United Kingdom, next only in frequency to cancer of the lung.

4 Predisposing factors are long-standing ulcerative colitis, pre-existing polyps, familial polyposis coli and hereditary non-polyposis colon cancer (HNPCC) genotype.

5 This is the commonest cause (in the United Kingdom) of a large bowel obstruction, either acute or chronic. A less common emergency is perforation, either into the general peritoneal cavity or locally, to form a pericolic abscess.

(See Chapter 25, *Lecture Notes on General Surgery.*)

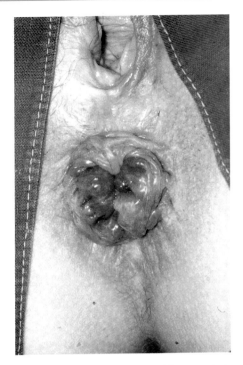

This photograph is of a 50-year-old woman in the lithotomy position immediately prior to surgery.

1 What condition is demonstrated?

2 What veins are involved and where do they drain?

3 What are her likely symptoms?

4 How would a carcinoma of the rectum have been excluded pre-operatively?

5 What serious local complication may occur in the early days following haemorrhoidectomy?

1 Third degree haemorrhoids—the piles (the two words are synonymous) remain persistently prolapsed outside the anal margin.

2 The superior haemorrhoidal veins, which drain into the inferior mesenteric vein, part of the portal venous system.

3 Rectal bleeding, prolapse and perhaps also mucous discharge and pruritus ani. Occasionally anaemia due to persistent bleeding.

4 A careful history, general physical examination including a rectal examination, sigmoidoscopy and, if indicated, a barium enema and colonoscopy.

5 Haemorrhage—usually on the same day, but occasionally delayed a week or so after surgery.

(See Chapter 26, *Lecture Notes on General Surgery.*)

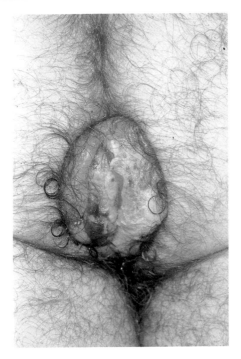

This man is suffering from an unpleasant complication of prolapsing piles.

1 What is this complication called?

2 What causes this?

3 From what symptoms will the patient suffer?

4 How is the patient managed conservatively?

5 What would be the outcome of this treatment, and is there an alternative, more radical therapy?

1 Thrombosed strangulated piles.

2 The prolapsing piles are gripped by the anal sphincter, the venous return is occluded and thrombosis occurs. Suppuration or ulceration may follow.

3 Acute anal pain with inability to reduce the piles.

4 Give opiate analgesia for the pain, elevate the foot of the bed and apply cold compresses.

5 The piles fibrose, often with complete or partial cure. However, this takes 2 or 3 weeks and many surgeons therefore advise an emergency haemorrhoidectomy.

(See Chapter 26, *Lecture Notes on General Surgery.*)

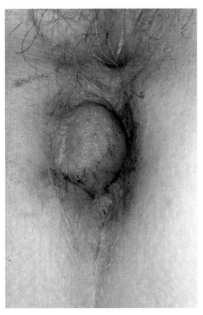 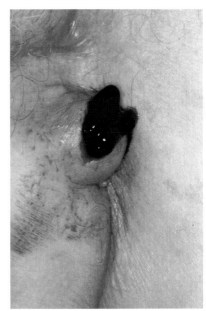

A   B

This patient presented with an acutely painful lump at the anal verge (A); (B) shows the operation performed that day under local anaesthesia.

1 What pathological condition is demonstrated in (A)?
2 What produces this?
3 Why is it so painful?
4 What happens if this lesion is left untreated?
5 What is the after-care and prognosis in this case?

1 A perianal haematoma.

2 Rupture of a tributary of the inferior haemorrhoidal plexus, often as a result of straining at stool.

3 The lower anal canal is supplied by a somatic innervation and is therefore sensitive to severe stretching.

4 It either slowly absorbs, leaving a fibrous skin tag, or may rupture spontaneously, discharging some clotted blood.

5 Hot baths are ordered and the small wound, where the haematoma has been evacuated, heals rapidly.

(See Chapter 26, *Lecture Notes on General Surgery*.)

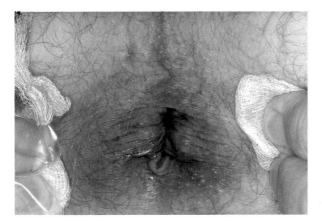

This patient's anal verge was examined under anaesthesia by pulling the buttocks apart.

1 What lesion can be seen at the 6 o'clock position?

2 What would be the characteristic symptoms of this?

3 What is meant by the 'sentinel pile', which is seen here?

4 Would you have been able to do a rectal examination on this patient in the clinic?

5 If multiple lesions such as this were seen at the anal verge, what underlying pathology would you suspect?

1 Anal fissure (fissure *in ano*).

2 Acute pain at the anal verge on defaecation, often accompanied by slight bleeding.

3 The torn tag of anal epithelium, which 'points' to the anal fissure.

4 Usually the anal sphincter is in spasm and it is far too painful to perform a rectal examination.

5 Crohn's disease of the large bowel.

(See Chapter 26, *Lecture Notes on General Surgery.*)

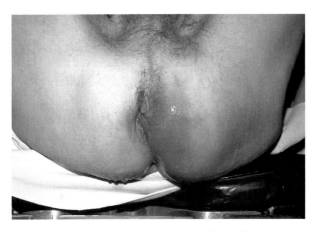

This patient presented with an acutely painful swelling to the left of the anal verge.

1 What is it called?

2 What is the definition of this condition?

3 What are the four classical features of this?

4 How should this be treated?

5 What complication may result from this condition in this particular location?

1 Perianal abscess.

2 An abscess is a localized collection of pus, usually, but not invariably, produced by pyogenic organisms.

3 Pain, swelling, redness and heat.

4 Surgical drainage.

5 A fistula *in ano* (see Question 78).

(See Chapter 26, *Lecture Notes on General Surgery*.)

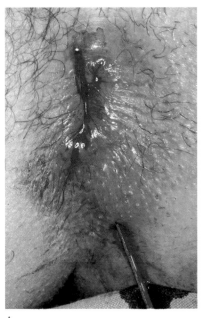

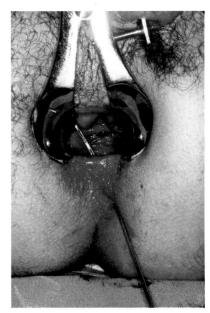

A

B

These two photographs were taken in the operating theatre. The patient was in the lithotomy position, under a general anaesthetic.

1 What pathology is demonstrated by the probe?

2 What is the precise definition of the term 'fistula'?

3 What typical symptoms might this patient have had?

4 What is the common underlying aetiology of this condition, and what are the rare causes?

5 What would be the surgical treatment for this particular patient?

1 A fistula *in ano*. The track runs from the perianal skin to open internally within the anal canal.

2 A fistula is an abnormal communication between two epithelial surfaces.

3 There is usually a story of an initial perianal abscess, which discharges. This is then followed by recurrent episodes of perianal infection with persistent discharge of pus.

4 The great majority result from an initial abscess forming in one of the anal glands, which discharges onto the perianal skin and into the anal canal. Rarely, fistulae are associated with Crohn's disease, ulcerative colitis, tuberculosis and carcinoma of the rectum.

5 The fistulous track is laid open and allowed to heal by granulation.

(See Chapter 26, *Lecture Notes on General Surgery*.)

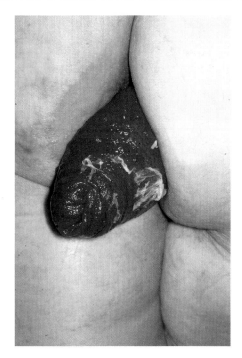

This photograph shows the anal region of a woman in her 70s.

1 What is the diagnosis?
2 Does this condition occur in men?
3 Can this occur in infants?
4 Apart from the discomfort, might the patient have any other symptoms?
5 If the patient is relatively fit, how should she be treated?

1 Complete rectal prolapse.

2 Usually it occurs in elderly women (often nulliparous) but it is found occasionally in men.

3 Partial (mucosal) prolapse may occur in healthy infants, but this usually is a self-curing condition.

4 Faecal incontinence due to stretching of the anal sphincter and mucous discharge from the prolapsed mucosa.

5 Surgical repair by fixing the rectum to the sacrum, e.g. by means of polyvinyl sponge, or mucosal resection by the Delorme's procedure.

(See Chapter 26, *Lecture Notes on General Surgery*.)

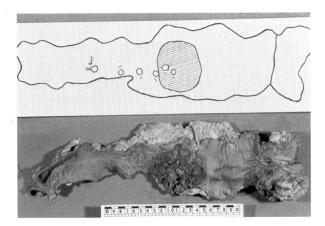

This rectum was removed by abdomino-perineal excision.

1 What pathology does it demonstrate?

2 What proportion of all large bowel lesions of this nature are found in the rectum?

3 What test would have been done to confirm the diagnosis before operation?

4 Where would this tumour spread to via the bloodstream?

5 Enumerate Dukes' classification of large bowel tumours.

1 Adenocarcinoma of the rectum.

2 One-third of all carcinomas of the large bowel occur within the rectum.

3 Sigmoidoscopy and histological examination of a biopsy specimen of the ulcer.

4 Via the portal vein to the liver and then to the lungs.

5 A: Confined to the rectal mucosa.

B: Penetrating the muscle wall.

C: Involving the regional lymph nodes.

D: Distal spread.

(See Chapter 26, *Lecture Notes on General Surgery*.)

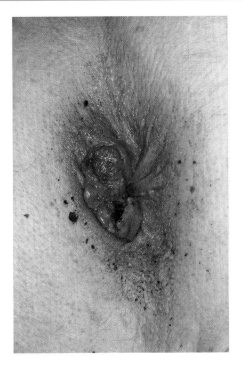

This man of 55 presented with a painful ulcerating tumour arising at the anal verge.

1 What is the histological type of epithelial tumour that originates at this site?

2 How would this clinical diagnosis be confirmed?

3 In contrast to the tumour shown in Question 80, where is the lymphatic spread from this growth?

4 What other malignant tumours may present at the anal verge?

5 This lesion is painful, whereas a comparable carcinoma of the rectum itself is not—how do you explain this?

1 Squamous carcinoma of the anal verge.

2 Biopsy and histological examination.

3 The inguinal nodes.

4 Downward spread from a carcinoma of the lower rectum, melanoma, basal cell carcinoma, carcinoid tumour and lymphoma.

5 The lower anal canal has a somatic innervation from the pudendal nerves, which transmit normal painful sensation. The rectum has an autonomic innervation, which will not register pain from a relatively small ulcerating lesion.

(See Chapter 26, *Lecture Notes on General Surgery*.)

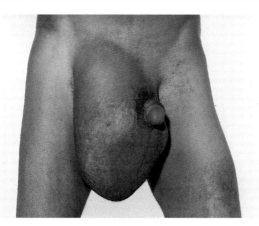

This man has noticed a lump in his right groin. It disappears over a few minutes when he lies down and gradually appears again when he stands.

1 What is the obvious diagnosis?

2 How often is this found in females?

3 Which anatomical structures do the contents of this swelling traverse?

4 What proportion occur on the right, on the left and bilaterally?

5 What serious emergency may complicate this lesion?

1 An indirect reducible right inguinal hernia.

2 Although much less common than in men, indirect inguinal hernias are not rare in females. Indeed, in women they are commoner than femoral hernias.

3 First the internal ring, then the inguinal canal and finally the external ring.

4 60% are on the right, 20% on the left and 20% are bilateral.

5 Strangulation, in which the contents of the hernia become constricted by the neck of the sac, gangrene being inevitable unless urgent surgery is performed.

(See Chapter 29, *Lecture Notes on General Surgery*.)

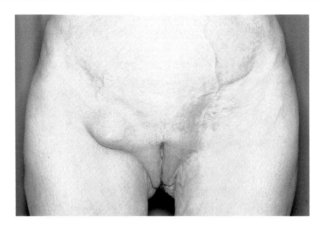

This is a photograph of the groins of an elderly woman.

1 What sort of hernia is shown on the right side?

2 Why is it more common in women than in men?

3 What is the important anatomical bony landmark used to differentiate this from an inguinal hernia?

4 Why is this hernia particularly dangerous?

5 What is meant by a Richter's hernia?

I Femoral hernia.

2 The pelvis is wider in the female than in the male; therefore the femoral canal is correspondingly larger.

3 The pubic tubercle. A femoral hernia is below and lateral to this, whereas an inguinal hernia passes above and medial to it.

4 The neck is narrow, so strangulation is a common complication.

5 Only part of the wall of the small intestine is caught up and strangulated.

(See Chapter 29, *Lecture Notes on General Surgery*.)

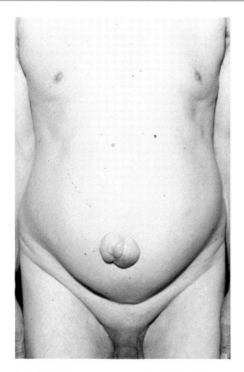

1 What is the correct name for this hernia?
2 What does it usually contain?
3 Is this hernia dangerous?
4 What is the condition that occurs at this site in children?
5 How does this differ from the adult form?

1 The correct name for this is a *para*-umbilical hernia, since these hernias occur just above or below the umbilicus and not directly through it.

2 Nearly always omentum and often, in addition, in large hernias, the transverse colon and small intestine.

3 Yes. The neck is narrow, and, like a femoral hernia, it is particularly prone to become irreducible or strangulated.

4 A congenital umbilical hernia, which results from failure of complete closure of the umbilical cicatrix.

5 The congenital umbilical hernia passes directly through the umbilicus. The vast majority close spontaneously during the first year of life and require no active treatment.

(See Chapter 29, *Lecture Notes on General Surgery*.)

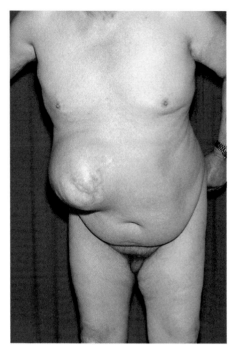

This patient noticed a bulge in his abdominal wall 6 months after a laparotomy. It has gradually enlarged since then.

1 What is this called?
2 Is it dangerous? If not, why not.
3 Classify its aetiological factors.
4 When would you advise surgical repair?
5 If not, what other treatment would you prescribe?

1 Incisional hernia.

2 No. It is usually wide necked and strangulation is, in consequence, rare.

3 (a) *Pre-operative* (e.g. uraemia, protein deficiency, vitamin C deficiency, jaundice, distension, chronic cough, etc.).

(b) *Operative* (poor technique, suture material of low tensile strength).

(c) *Post-operative* (e.g. cough, abdominal distension, wound infection or haematoma).

4 If the patient's general condition is good and the hernia is troubling him, surgical repair of the hernia is advised.

5 If operation is considered inadvisable, prescribe an abdominal belt.

(See Chapter 29, *Lecture Notes on General Surgery*.)

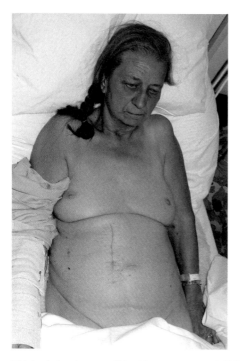

This is obviously a very ill-looking woman, aged 65. The scar on her abdomen is where she had recently undergone a by-pass for an extensive obstructing carcinoma of the pylorus.

1 What is the biochemical explanation of her colour change?
2 Classify the three large groups of causes of this condition.
3 Which of these three groups usually only produces a tinge of jaundice?
4 What is the likely cause of the jaundice in this patient?
5 This patient has a prolonged prothrombin time. Why?

1 Jaundice is due to staining of the tissues with bilirubin. It becomes clinically detectable when the serum level rises to over 35 μmol/l.

2 The causes of jaundice are classified into:

(a) *Pre-hepatic* (haemolytic disorders).

(b) *Hepatic*: due to liver disease or destruction.

(c) *Post-hepatic*: obstruction within the lumen (e.g. gall stones), in the wall (e.g. congenital, traumatic stricture, bile duct tumour) or external compression of the duct (e.g. tumours of pancreas, pancreatitis).

3 Pre-hepatic jaundice, where the bilirubin is rarely raised higher than 100 μmol/l. Since the ducts are not obstructed, large amounts of excess bilirubin are excreted into the gut.

4 She is likely to have developed liver secondaries from her gastric primary.

5 Vitamin K, necessary for prothrombin synthesis, is fat soluble and requires bile salts for its absorption into the gut. In addition, extensive liver damage from her secondary deposits may prevent hepatic synthesis of prothrombin.

(See Chapter 30, *Lecture Notes on General Surgery*.)

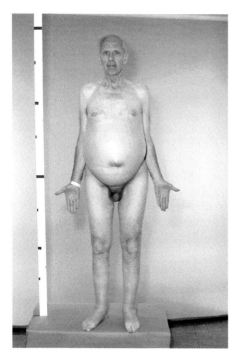

This patient is an alcoholic. He presented with slight clinical jaundice, gross ascites and pitting oedema of the legs.

1 What is the likely diagnosis?
2 What factors are responsible for the ascites?
3 What do you notice at the umbilicus?
4 What CNS effects would you look for in such a patient?
5 What can be done to relieve the ascites?

1 Alcoholic cirrhosis.

2 Ascites is here due to a combination of factors—raised portal pressure, low serum albumin, increased aldosterone (due to liver damage) with sodium retention, and increased hepatic lymphatic pressure.

3 An umbilical hernia—a common finding in the grossly distended abdomen.

4 Mental changes, flapping tremor and hepatic coma (portal-systemic encephalopathy).

5 A low sodium, high protein diet and diuretics, peritoneovenous shunt in severe and refractory cases.

(See Chapter 30, *Lecture Notes on General Surgery*.)

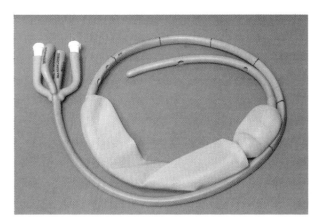

This instrument is used in the emergency treatment of certain cases of severe haematemesis.

1 What is it called?

2 For what source of haematemesis is it employed?

3 How does it control the haemorrhage in these cases?

4 What is the purpose of the narrow distal end of the tube, which leads into the stomach?

5 What injection technique can be used to deal with this source of haemorrhage?

1 Sengstaken tube.

2 Bleeding oesophageal and gastric varices in portal hypertension.

3 The balloons in the oesophagus and in the cardia are blown up and compress the varices.

4 The gastric tube is used for aspirating the stomach or for feeding purposes.

5 The varices can be injected through a fibreoptic oesophagoscope using sclerosing fluid.

(See Chapter 30, *Lecture Notes on General Surgery*.)

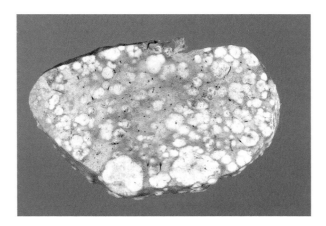

This is a slice through a liver at post-mortem.

1 Describe what you can see.

2 What is this appearance due to?

3 What is the description of the characteristic cut surface of these lesions and what produces this appearance?

4 List the common primary sites for the origin of these lesions in the United Kingdom.

5 How often will these lesions be found at post-mortem on patients dying of malignant disease?

1 The liver is almost replaced by widespread whitish deposits.

2 Extensive blood-borne metastases.

3 The cut surface classically has the umbilicated appearance due to necrosis in the centre of the deposits.

4 Large bowel, stomach, lung and breast account for the majority of cases, although carcinomas at any site and malignant melanoma may all metastasize to the liver.

5 In one-third of cases.

(See Chapter 30, *Lecture Notes on General Surgery*.)

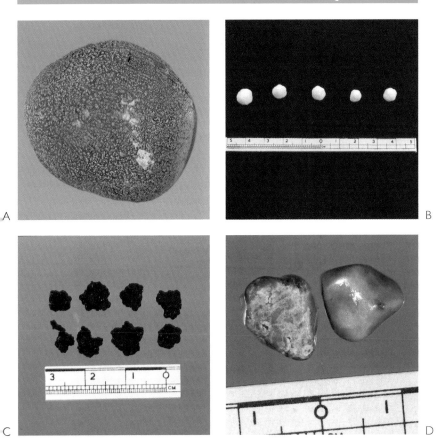

A

B

C

D

These are examples of gall stones removed from four different patients at cholecystectomy.

1 Name the principal constituents of the calculi shown in (A), (B), (C) and (D).

2 What are the other names commonly given to the stones shown in (A), (B) and (D)?

3 If the stones shown in (A) and (D) were cut open, what would be the appearances of their cut surfaces?

4 Cholesterol is insoluble in water; what is the mechanism that keeps it in solution in bile? What relationship has this got with the aetiology of cholesterol-containing stones?

5 What associated diseases may be found in patients who develop stones (C)?

1 (A) Cholesterol.

   (B) Cholesterol.

   (C) Bile pigment.

   (D) Mixed cholesterol and bile pigment.

2 (A) Cholesterol 'solitaire'.

   (B) 'Mulberry' stones.

   (D) Faceted stones.

3 (A) Demonstrates radiating cholesterol crystals.

   (D) Shows concentric rings of bile pigment and cholesterol.

4 Cholesterol is held in solution in the bile as a mixed micelle with bile salts and phospholipids. The bile from patients with cholesterol-containing stones shows a reduction in concentration of both these substances in relation to the cholesterol content, which favours cholesterol crystallization ('lithogenic bile').

5 Pigment stones occur particularly in patients with haemolytic anaemias, e.g. acholuric jaundice, where excess of circulating bile pigment is deposited in the biliary tract.

(See Chapter 31, *Lecture Notes on General Surgery*.)

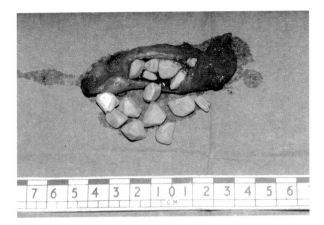

This is a specimen of a gall bladder removed at cholecystectomy.

1 What does it contain?

2 What does its wall demonstrate?

3 What are the typical features of biliary colic?

4 What physical signs might you have elicited on this patient's admission to hospital?

5 What is the least disturbing special investigation in such a case?

1 Multiple mixed (cholesterol and bile pigment) gall stones.

2 The gall bladder wall is acutely inflamed — acute cholecystitis.

3 The pain is severe, usually situated in the right subcostal region; but may be epigastric or spread as a band across the upper abdomen. Radiation to the lower pole of the right scapula is common. Characteristically the patient is restless and rolls about in agony. Often there is associated vomiting and sweating.

4 The patient has a pyrexia and may be toxic. The upper abdomen would be extremely tender and there may be a palpable mass in the region of the gall bladder. Look for jaundice and test the urine for bile.

5 An ultrasound of the upper abdomen is very accurate in revealing gall stones, as well as being safe and painless. These are demonstrated as intensely echogenic foci, which cast a characteristic 'shadow'.

(See Chapter 31, *Lecture Notes on General Surgery*.)

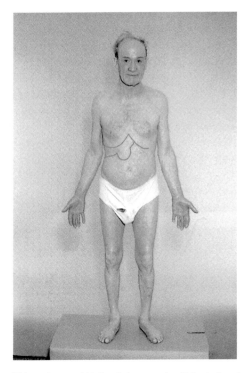

This patient and his family have noticed his obvious jaundice, but he has experienced no pain. The physical signs elicited on abdominal examination have been outlined with a skin marker.

1 What physical signs are demonstrated?

2 What is the name of the law based on these physical signs?

3 What conclusions can you deduce from these findings?

4 In view of the absence of pain, what type of pancreatic tumour may this patient have?

5 What physical sign can you see on his underpants?

1 The liver is enlarged and a distended gall bladder can be detected.

2 Courvoisier's law.

3 In the presence of jaundice, if the gall bladder is palpable, then the jaundice is unlikely to be due to stone (and, therefore, likely to be due to a carcinoma of the pancreas).

4 The absence of pain suggests that the tumour is in the region of the ampulla. This will produce early obstruction of the bile duct, before extensive painful invasion of the surrounding tissues has taken place.

5 He has dribbled some urine onto his underpants; this has evaporated leaving a stain of bilirubin. Obviously he has bilirubinuria!

(See Chapters 31 and 32, *Lecture Notes on General Surgery*.)

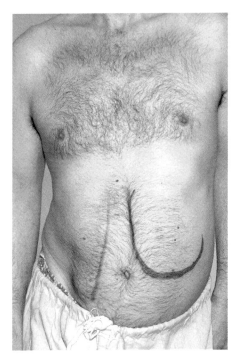

This man had a laparotomy for acute abdominal pain, at which time acute pancreatitis was diagnosed. Subsequently he gradually developed this enormous but painless cystic mass in the upper abdomen.

1 What is the diagnosis?
2 What produces this?
3 What would be the percussion note over such a mass?
4 What special investigations are useful in delineating this mass?
5 How are such cysts treated?

1 Pancreatic pseudocyst.

2 An effusion of pancreatic secretions into the lesser sac of the peritoneum.

3 When small, the cyst is retroperitoneal and is apparently resonant because of the loops of gas-filled bowel and stomach in front of it. As it increases in size, the intestine is pushed away and the mass becomes dull to percussion, as in this case.

4 It may be demonstrated by ultrasonography, but the cyst may be obscured by gas in the upper gastrointestinal tract. CT scanning may be more valuable.

5 It may often be possible to aspirate the cyst percutaneously under ultrasound or CT scan control. If not, the cyst is drained internally by anastomosis either to the posterior wall of the stomach or to the small intestine.

(See Chapter 32, *Lecture Notes on General Surgery*.)

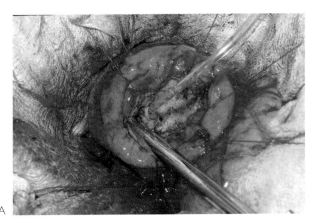

A

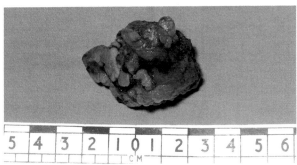

B

A man of 70 presented with painless progressive jaundice. Courvoisier's sign (see Question 92) was positive; (A) demonstrates the operative findings — the second part of the duodenum has been opened and an ulcerated mass exposed; (B) shows the excised tumour.

1 What is this tumour and from which structures may it have originated?

2 Why was the patient's jaundice painless?

3 What is the distribution of carcinoma in the head, the body and the tail of the pancreas?

4 What is the age and sex distribution of pancreatic carcinoma, and what is apparently happening to its incidence?

5 In this patient, an incontrovertible diagnosis was established before his laparotomy. How was this achieved?

I This is a periampullary carcinoma. It may arise from the ampulla of Vater, the lower end of the common bile duct or the adjacent duodenal mucosa.

2 The periampullary carcinoma compresses the lower end of the common bile duct and produces jaundice before there is extensive painful invasion of surrounding tissues by the tumour.

3 Carcinoma of the pancreas occurs most commonly in the head of the pancreas, then in the body and then in the tail. The distribution is approximately 60%, 25% and 15%, respectively.

4 The disease occurs particularly in middle-aged and elderly subjects. Males are affected twice as commonly as females. The incidence of the tumour is apparently increasing, perhaps because of the rising age of the population and perhaps also because of the more sophisticated techniques of diagnosis.

5 This patient underwent pre-operative fibreoptic endoscopy. The tumour was visualized in the second part of the duodenum and a positive biopsy obtained.

(See Chapter 32, *Lecture Notes on General Surgery*.)

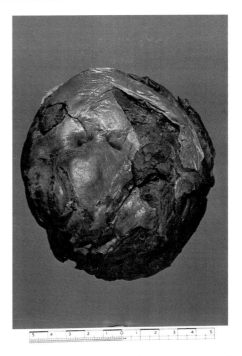

This is the spleen removed as an emergency from a young man who was involved in a motor cycle accident.

1 What is the obvious pathology?

2 What is meant by 'delayed rupture of the spleen'?

3 What is meant by 'spontaneous rupture of the spleen'?

4 What physical signs might you have elicited in the examination of this patient's abdomen?

5 What general clinical features would have suggested profound blood loss?

1 Extensive lacerations of the spleen.

2 Delayed rupture may occur hours or even several days after trauma. A sub-capsular haematoma forms, which increases in size and then suddenly ruptures.

3 A spleen diseased by malaria, glandular fever, leukaemia, etc. may rupture after only trivial trauma.

4 The abdomen is generally tender, particularly on the left side, but rigidity may vary from being generalized and extreme to being confined to only slight guarding in the left flank. The percussion note is impaired in the left flank due to the local collection of blood.

5 The patient is pale, cold and sweating. There is progressive fall in the blood pressure and a progressive rise in the pulse rate.

(See Chapter 33, *Lecture Notes on General Surgery.*)

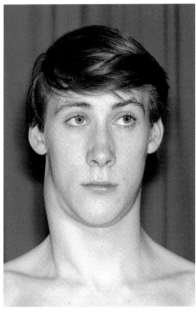

A

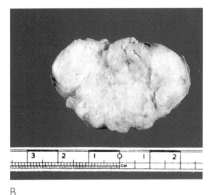

B

This young man presented with a painless mass of discrete, rubbery lymph nodes in the right side of the neck (A). These have progressively enlarged over the past several months. (B) shows a cross-section through the surgically excised specimen.

1 What steps would you have taken in your clinical examination of the patient to try and establish the cause of his lymphadenopathy?

2 If all your findings, apart from these enlarged cervical nodes, had been negative, what would have been your provisional clinical diagnosis?

3 What special investigations would you have then ordered?

4 Describe the macroscopic appearance of the excised nodes in (B).

5 Histologically, this proved to be Hodgkin's disease. What is the name of the typical cells seen under the microscope in this condition?

I (a) Search the area drained by the involved lymph nodes for a possible primary source of infection or malignant disease; in this instance, a careful examination of the head, neck and throat.

(b) Examine the other lymph node areas to determine if there is a generalized lymphadenopathy.

(c) Examine the abdomen for splenomegaly and hepatomegaly; their enlargement would suggest lymphoma, lymphatic leukaemia, sarcoid or glandular fever.

2 Hodgkin's disease or non-Hodgkin's lymphoma.

3 (a) Examination of a blood film (glandular fever, lymphatic leukaemia).

(b) Chest X-ray (may reveal evidence of enlarged mediastinal nodes or a primary occult tumour). The X-ray may also demonstrate if the cervical lymph nodes show the typical spotty calcification of tuberculosis.

(c) Biopsy to establish definite histological proof of the diagnosis.

4 The lymph nodes show diffuse infiltration and are discrete — macroscopically consistent with a diagnosis of a lymphoma.

5 Dorothy Reed giant cells.

(See Chapter 34, *Lecture Notes on General Surgery.*)

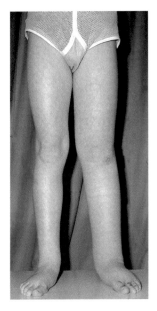

This woman, aged 21, has had swollen legs since the age of 14 years. She is otherwise extremely fit.

1 What is this condition called?

2 What is its aetiology?

3 What name is given to the familial variety of this disease?

4 Methylene blue has been injected subcutaneously into the dorsum of the left foot the day before. What do you notice?

5 How is this condition treated?

1 Lymphoedema—in full, lymphoedema praecox, since it commenced at puberty.

2 Congenital abnormality of the lymphatic channels of the lower limbs.

3 Milroy's disease.

4 It has persisted, thus confirming the virtual absence of lymphatic drainage.

5 Elevation of the lower limbs at night together with firm elastic bandaging. Surgical excision is only carried out in gross cases.

(See Chapter 34, *Lecture Notes on General Surgery*.)

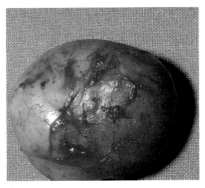

A

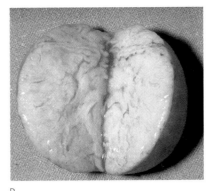

B

This lump was enucleated from the breast of a girl of 17 years. (A) shows its intact appearance, and (B) shows its cut surface.

1 What is the diagnosis?
2 Describe the naked eye appearance of the tumour.
3 What is its microscopic appearance?
4 What are the physical signs in a typical case?
5 Can this tumour occur in post-menopausal women?

1 Fibroadenoma of the breast.

2 An encapsulated tumour with a whorled appearance on its cut surface.

3 Fibrous tissue surrounding epithelial duct proliferation.

4 A highly mobile, non-attached lump in the breast—the so-called 'breast mouse'.

5 Rarely the condition is found in middle-aged or elderly women, although it is much commoner in teenagers and in the early 20s.

(See Chapter 35, *Lecture Notes on General Surgery*.)

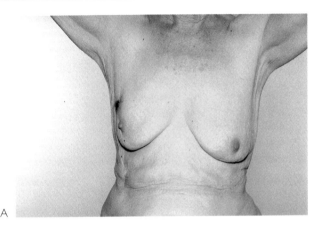

A

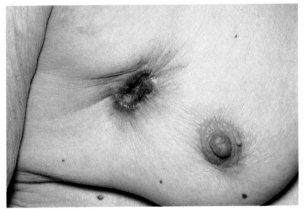

B

These photographs show a general and a close-up view of the breast of a woman aged 75.

1 What are the signs that you can see of an obvious carcinoma of the breast?

2 How common is breast cancer in the United Kingdom?

3 How often is it found in male subjects?

4 Where would you examine this patient clinically for evidence of dissemination of the tumour?

5 Is there anything known about predisposing factors or aetiology in this disease?

1 The right nipple is elevated compared with the left. There is a malignant ulcer in the upper outer quadrant of the breast, with typical raised edges and puckering of the surrounding skin.

2 This is the commonest killing cancer of women, and accounts for about 15 000 deaths annually in England and Wales.

3 About 1% of all cancers of the breast occur in men.

4 (a) *Lymphatic spread*: examine the axillary and supraclavicular nodes.

(b) *Blood spread*: examine the liver, lungs, bony skeleton, and CNS.

(c) *Transcoelomic spread*: examine for ascites and pleural effusion.

5 Very little is known about aetiology or predisposing factors. There is a family tendency, it is rare in the Far East and it is less likely to affect women who have had pregnancies in their teens. Carriage of the BRCA1 and BRCA2 genes are significant risk factors.

(See Chapter 35, *Lecture Notes on General Surgery*.)

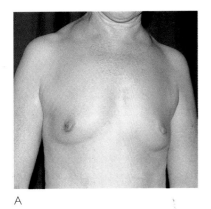

A

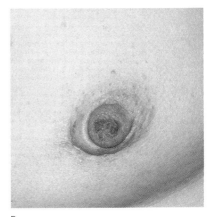

B

This 60-year-old woman complained of unilateral 'sore' right nipple shown in (A); (B) is a close-up view of this.

1 What is your clinical diagnosis?

2 What are the typical clinical features of this condition?

3 What are two other diseases that bear this surgeon's name?

4 What are the diagnostic findings on microscopic examination of a biopsy of this nipple?

5 What is the commonly held theory of the aetiology of this disease?

1 Paget's disease of the nipple.

2 A unilateral, red, bleeding, eczematous lesion of the nipple, which is eventually destroyed by the disease. There may or may not be a palpable underlying carcinoma.

3 Paget's disease of the bone and Paget's disease of the penis (carcinoma *in situ*).

4 The deep layers of the epithelium contain multiple, clear Paget cells with small dark nuclei. The underlying dermis contains an inflammatory cellular infiltration. There is usually an associated intraduct carcinoma.

5 Paget's disease probably represents the invasion of the nipple by malignant cells arising in a mammary duct, which also give origin to the associated breast tumour.

(See Chapter 35, *Lecture Notes on General Surgery*.)

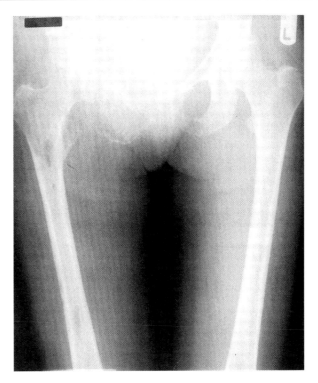

This is the X-ray of a woman aged 50 years. Two years previously she had undergone a right mastectomy for carcinoma of the breast. She now complains of severe pain in the region of the right hip.

1 Describe the lesions you can see on this X-ray.

2 What is the diagnosis?

3 Where else would you expect to find bony secondaries, and why?

4 What other tumours commonly metastasize to bone?

5 Where else might you commonly find blood-borne metastases from carcinoma of the breast?

1 There are extensive lytic lesions in the right femoral neck, the trochanters and femoral shaft. Further lytic areas are seen in the right pubis, where there is a pathological fracture of the upper ramus. Less extensive lytic areas are seen in the public bone on the left side.

2 Osteolytic secondaries from the breast carcinoma.

3 Bony deposits occur at the sites of red bone marrow — skull, vertebrae, ribs, sternum and upper end of the humerus, as well as in the pelvis and femur, as shown in this X-ray.

4 Carcinoma of lung, prostate, kidney and thyroid, together with the breast, are the five tumours that commonly produce bony secondaries (see Question 119).

5 Apart from bone, blood-borne deposits from carcinoma of the breast occur especially in the lungs and liver. The brain, ovaries and suprarenals are also frequent foci of deposits.

(See Chapter 35, *Lecture Notes on General Surgery*.)

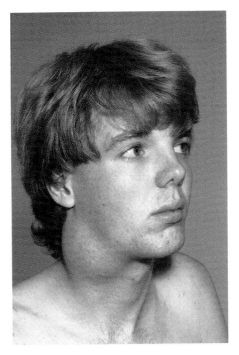

This teenager presented with a slowly enlarging, painless, cystic swelling in the neck.

1 What is the likely diagnosis?
2 What is the embryological explanation of this cyst?
3 What material does it contain?
4 What complication may it undergo?
5 What differential diagnoses would you have to consider?

1 A branchial cyst.

2 The second branchial arch in the fetus grows down over the third and fourth arches to form the cervical sinus. This usually disappears but its persistence is believed to lead to the formation of a branchial cyst, sinus or fistula.

3 The fluid looks like pus but actually consists of cholesterol crystals.

4 The branchial cyst may become infected and may discharge as a branchial sinus.

5 Tuberculous cervical nodes or, if infected, an acute lymphadenitis.

(See Chapter 36, *Lecture Notes on General Surgery*.)

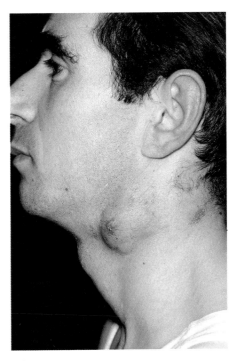

This young immigrant presented with a relatively painless abscess in the neck. On palpation, the skin over it shows no evidence of increased heat — it was a 'cold abscess'.

1 What is your clinical diagnosis?
2 In what racial groups would you consider this possibility?
3 What would be the differential diagnoses?
4 At operation, the infected lymph node had broken through the deep fascia and the abscess lay in the subcutaneous tissues. What is this type of abscess called?
5 What would happen if the abscess was left untreated?

1 Tuberculous cervical adenitis with an overlying abscess.

2 Immigrants from Third World countries where tuberculosis is still common.

3 Acute lymphadenitis (which feels hot and which is particularly painful and tender); branchial cyst.

4 A 'collar stud' abscess.

5 The abscess will discharge onto the skin, resulting in a chronic tuberculous sinus.

(See Chapter 36, *Lecture Notes on General Surgery*.)

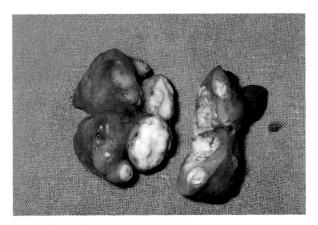

This is a mass of cervical lymph nodes excised from a girl of 14, a recent immigrant from the Indian subcontinent.

1 What is the diagnosis?

2 What is the name given to this typical pus — and why?

3 What may well have been seen on a pre-operative X-ray of this girl's neck?

4 What was the probable pathway of the tuberculous organisms into these nodes?

5 Outline the treatment of this condition.

1 Tuberculous cervical adenitis.

2 Caseous pus—the word means 'cheesy', because of its resemblance to cream cheese.

3 Chronic tuberculous nodes usually show flecks of calcification.

4 Cervical nodes are usually secondarily involved from a tonsillar primary focus. The organisms may be human or bovine (the latter from infected milk).

5 Enlarged nodes should be excised (as in this case). If the patient presents with a 'collar stud' abscess (see Question 103), the pus is evacuated, a search made for the hole penetrating through the deep fascia, and the underlying caseating node evacuated by curettage. Operative treatment should be combined with antituberculous chemotherapy.

(See Chapter 36, *Lecture Notes on General Surgery*.)

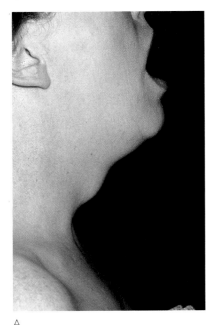

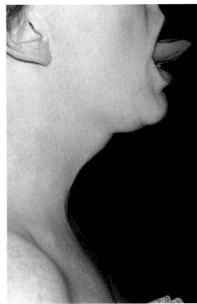

A   B

This young woman has a lump in the neck, which moves on swallowing.

1 What physical sign is being demonstrated in these two photographs?

2 What is the diagnosis?

3 What is the embryological explanation of this physical sign?

4 What other congenital anomalies may result from this embryological process of development?

5 What is the treatment for this swelling?

1 The lump moves upwards when the patient protrudes her tongue.

2 Thyroglossal cyst.

3 The thyroid develops from the foramen caecum at the base of the tongue and descends to its definitive position. The cyst forms in embryological remnants of the thyroid and the tract retains its attachment to the base of the tongue. It moves on swallowing because of its attachment to the larynx by the pretracheal fascia.

4 Lingual thyroid; thyroglossal fistula; pyramidal lobe attached to the isthmus of the thyroid; and a retrosternal thyroid, when the thyroid descends beyond its normal station into the superior mediastinum.

5 A preliminary radio-iodine scan should be performed to ensure that there is normal thyroid tissue present in the correct place, after which the cyst is removed surgically.

(See Chapter 37, *Lecture Notes of General Surgery*.)

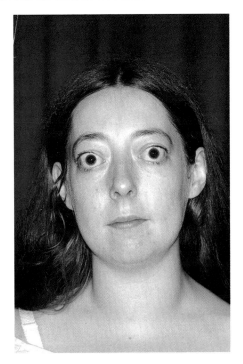

This girl's endocrine disease can be diagnosed at a glance.
1 What is the diagnosis?
2 This girl's thyroid is smoothly enlarged. Is thyroid hypertrophy invariable in this disease?
3 What changes within the orbit produce the eye signs?
4 What may occur in very advanced stages of exophthalmos?
5 What are the cardiovascular features that may occur in this disease?

I Grave's disease or primary hyperthyroidism.

2 Although the thyroid is usually enlarged in this condition it is not invariably so.

3 Exophthalmos is produced by oedema and actual increase in the mass of the orbital fat and extrinsic muscles of the eye. The aetiology is unknown.

4 If the exophthalmos is severe, the extrinsic muscles of the eye may be damaged, resulting in incoordination or paralysis of eye movement (exophthalmic ophthalmoplegia). If the patient is unable to close her eyelids, corneal ulceration may develop.

5 Tachycardia and an elevated sleeping pulse rate. There may be atrial fibrillation and the patient may develop heart failure.

(See Chapter 37, *Lecture Notes on General Surgery.*)

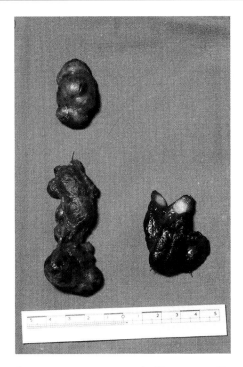

A young woman presented with a mass of lymph nodes in the right side of the neck. After biopsy, she was submitted to excision of these lymph nodes together with removal of the right lobe of the thyroid.

1 What does the specimen demonstrate?
2 What is the likely histology of the white nodule in the thyroid?
3 Enumerate the other types of primary carcinoma of the thyroid.
4 What is the sex distribution of these tumours?
5 What is the bloodstream spread of thyroid carcinoma?

215

1 There is a small nodule of tumour in the upper pole of the thyroid lobe. The removed lymph nodes are grossly enlarged and must obviously be invaded by secondary deposits.

2 A papillary carcinoma of the thyroid may typically produce deposits in the lymph nodes and only a careful search of the thyroid gland will reveal a well-differentiated tumour in the lobe on that side.

3 The other carcinomas are:

(a) Follicular (usually in young and middle-aged adults).

(b) Medullary (arising from the parafollicular cells).

(c) Anaplastic (usually in the elderly).

4 Medullary carcinoma has a roughly equal sex distribution. The other carcinomas affect females twice as often as males.

5 Bloodstream spread occurs to the lungs and brain. It is one of the tumours that commonly produces bony secondary deposits (see Question 119).

(See Chapter 37, *Lecture Notes on General Surgery.*)

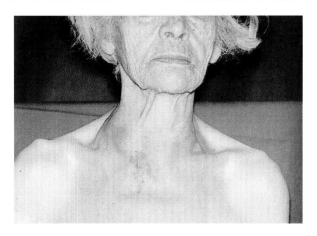

This elderly woman presented with a rapidly enlarging hard mass in the neck, which moves on swallowing. She has also recently lost her voice.

1 What is the clinical diagnosis?

2 What is its likely histology, and why is this anomalous when compared with most tumours at other sites?

3 Why has she lost her voice?

4 How could you confirm this as the cause?

5 What treatment might be possible in her case?

1 This large invasive mass is obviously a carcinoma of the thyroid.

2 Rapidly enlarging thyroid cancers in the elderly are usually anaplastic carcinomas. This is the reversal of the state of affairs in other organs, in that the more malignant tumours of the thyroid occur in the older age group.

3 Invasion of the recurrent laryngeal nerve on one or both sides.

4 The vocal cords are inspected by indirect laryngoscopy. The paralysed cord will be immobile when the patient attempts to phonate.

5 This extensive tumour is already invading the recurrent laryngeal nerve (hence the loss of voice) and is beyond treatment by radical thyroidectomy. Palliative radiotherapy may give temporary relief and a tracheostomy may eventually be required for the obstructed airway.

(See Chapter 37, *Lecture Notes on General Surgery*.)

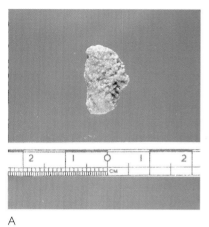

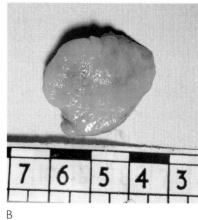

A   B

(A) demonstrates the calcium oxalate stone removed from the pelvi-ureteric junction of a young man aged 24 years; (B) shows the lesion that was removed from his neck 2 weeks later. The second pathology is directly linked to the development of the first.

1 What is the lesion shown in (B)?

2 What biochemical investigation on the patient's serum would have made one suspect this condition to be present?

3 List other causes of a raised serum calcium.

4 What screening technique may be used to visualize this neck lesion pre-operatively?

5 What other endocrine tumours may co-exist with this tumour, and what is the syndrome called when this occurs?

1 A parathyroid adenoma.

2 The serum calcium is usually raised to above 2.75 mmol/l (in addition the serum phosphate level is low).

3 Other causes of a raised serum calcium include metastatic cancer (particularly of the breast), multiple myeloma, sarcoidosis and the milk alkali syndrome.

4 The most efficient non-invasive scanning technique is first to perform a technetium scan of the neck. Technetium is taken up specifically by the thyroid. This is followed by a thallium scan, which is taken up by both the thyroid and the parathyroid. Subtraction of the first scan from the second reveals a 'hot spot', which denotes a functioning parathyroid tumour.

5 A parathyroid adenoma may co-exist with other endocrine tumours — pancreatic islet cell tumour, anterior pituitary adenoma, medullary carcinoma of the thyroid and phaeochromocytoma of the suprarenal medulla (the multiple endocrine adenoma syndrome).

(See Chapter 38, *Lecture Notes on General Surgery*.)

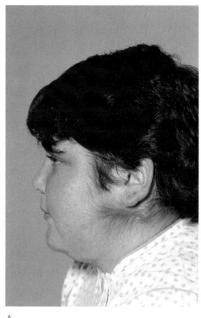

A

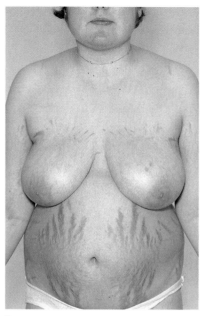

B

This young girl went to her general practitioner complaining of excessive growth of hair on her face.

1 What is the eponymous name of the endocrine disease from which she is suffering?

2 What is the cause of this condition?

3 Describe the appearances of her abdomen in (B).

4 What bone changes may occur in this disease?

5 What laboratory examination of her urine would confirm your clinical diagnosis?

1 Cushing's syndrome.

2 Oversecretion of suprarenal corticosteroids.

3 The abdomen is obese (she demonstrates the characteristic central distribution of her obesity) and there are prominent abdominal striae.

4 Osteoporosis.

5 The urinary ketosteroid level is raised and rises still further in cases of suprarenal hyperplasia following the additional stimulation of ACTH. Failure of the level to rise on ACTH suggests a suprarenal autonomous tumour rather than simple hyperplasia.

(See Chapter 40, *Lecture Notes on General Surgery*.)

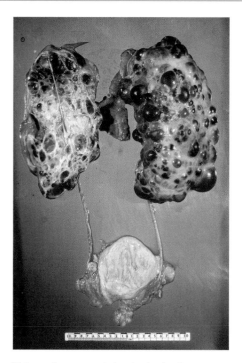

This specimen was obviously obtained at post-mortem!

1 What is the diagnosis and what is its embryological explanation?
2 Is it an inherited disease?
3 How may this condition present?
4 What are the common causes of death from this condition?
5 How may it be treated?

1 Polycystic disease of the kidneys. It is believed to be due to failure of fusion of tubules of the metanephros with the metanephric duct.

2 Yes. It is inherited either as an autosomal dominant (adult) or autosomal recessive (paediatric) disease.

3 (a) At birth — obstructed labour.

   (b) Infancy — death from multiple congenital abnormalities.

   (c) Young adults — symptomless bilateral renal masses.

   (d) Haematuria, loin pain and renal infection.

   (e) Hypertension, often presenting in a young adult.

   (f) Renal failure.

4 The patient may die either from renal failure or from the complications of hypertension (cardiac failure or stroke).

5 Renal transplantation.

(See Chapter 41, *Lecture Notes on General Surgery*.)

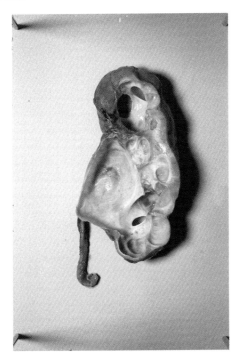

This almost functionless kidney was removed at nephrectomy. The pelvis and calyces show gross dilatation and there is considerable destruction of the renal substance.

1 What term is applied to this condition?
2 What are the causes of this pathology?
3 List its common complications.
4 What special investigations are used to demonstrate this condition?
5 Outline its treatment.

1 Hydronephrosis.

2 This may result either from congenital neuromuscular incoordination at the pelvi-ureteric junction or from obstruction along the urinary tract (e.g. ureteric stone or prostatic obstruction).

3 (a) Infection, resulting in pyonephrosis.

(b) Stone formation.

(c) Hypertension.

(d) Uraemia, where there is extensive bilateral disease.

(e) Traumatic rupture.

4 An intravenous urogram may demonstrate the enlarged renal pelvis and the dilated club-like calyces. If renal function is severely impaired the kidney may not secrete the contrast. In such a case the hydronephrosis can be demonstrated by ultrasonography or a CT scan.

5 Remove any underlying obstructive cause. If the aetiology is neuromuscular incoordination, a plastic operation is performed at the pelvi-ureteric junction. A completely useless (particularly an infected) kidney is an indication for nephrectomy, provided the other kidney has reasonable function.

(See Chapter 41, *Lecture Notes on General Surgery.*)

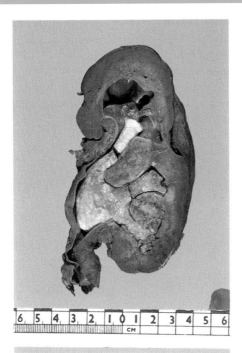

This kidney was removed at nephrectomy.

1 Describe the pathology it demonstrates.
2 What is the name given to the calculus?
3 What is its chemical composition?
4 What will be the likely findings in this patient's urine?
5 What would an intravenous pyelogram have demonstrated in this case?

1 The pelvis is grossly dilated and inflamed—a pyonephrosis. There is considerable destruction of the renal substance. The pelvis contains a large calculus.

2 A stag horn calculus.

3 Calcium, ammonium and magnesium phosphate ('triple phosphate stone').

4 If the ureter is completely obstructed there may be little to find on examining the urine although more commonly pyuria is a marked feature. The infecting organism is *E. coli* in the majority of cases.

5 An intravenous urogram shows little or no function. The enlarged renal shadow is usually obvious. Because of its high content of calcium, the stone is easily visible on the preliminary plain film of the abdomen.

(See Chapter 41, *Lecture Notes on General Surgery.*)

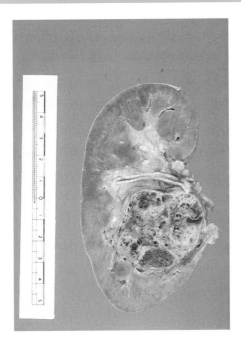

This is the cut section of a kidney that has been removed surgically.

1 What are the names given to this tumour?

2 What is its microscopic appearance?

3 What are the local symptoms, which may draw attention to its presence?

4 In what other ways may it present?

5 Describe how the tumour may metastasize.

1 Adenocarcinoma is the most accurate term. 'Hypernephroma' is an archaic term dating back to the theory of its origin from suprarenal rests postulated by Grawitz, whose name is also applied eponymously to this disease.

2 Microscopically the tumour cells are typically large, with abundant foamy cytoplasm and with a small central densely staining nucleus—the so-called 'clear cell tumour'.

3 40% present with haematuria and the bleeding may produce clot colic. Another 40% of patients present with a mass or an aching pain in the loin.

4 The remaining 20% of patients manifest either with secondary deposits (e.g. a pathological fracture) or with the general features of malignant disease (anaemia and loss of weight). Occasionally the tumour presents with a pyrexia of unknown origin.

5 By lymphatic spread to the para-aortic lymph nodes, and by bloodstream dissemination along the renal vein into the inferior vena cava, and thence to the lungs, skeleton, brain and elsewhere.

(See Chapter 41, *Lecture Notes on General Surgery.*)

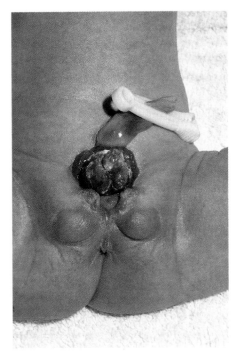

This is the appearance of the abdomen of a newborn girl.

1 What is the name of this condition?

2 What is the nature of this abnormality?

3 This child has the commonly associated abnormality of the pelvic girdle (the visible nodule on each side is the corresponding pubic ramus) — what does this comprise?

4 Left untreated, what is the natural history of this condition?

5 What surgical treatment is usually carried out?

I Ectopia vesicae.

2 The bladder fails to develop properly and the ureters, together with the bladder trigone, open directly onto the anterior abdominal wall. In the male there is an associated epispadias of the penis.

3 Frequently (as in this case) there is maldevelopment of the pubic bones with a failure of the pubes to meet at the symphysis. This results in a widened pelvis and the child walks with a waddling gait.

4 The child may die of pyelonephritis due to ascending infection. Carcinoma of the bladder rudiment may develop after initial metaplastic change.

5 Attempts to reconstruct the bladder are usually unsuccessful. Treatment usually comprises reimplantation of the ureters into an ileal conduit, with excision of the bladder remnant as a prophylaxis against malignant change.

(See Chapter 42, *Lecture Notes on General Surgery*.)

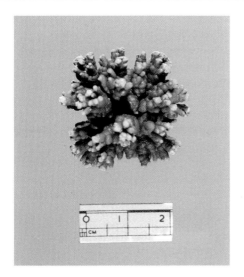

This large, sharp, spiky calculus was removed from the bladder of a man aged 62 years.

1 What is its chemical composition?
2 What accounts for its colour?
3 What is the classical triad of symptoms produced by a bladder stone?
4 What special investigations are used to confirm the clinical diagnosis of a bladder stone?
5 Name the two other common varieties of calculus of the urinary tract.

1 This spiky appearance is typical of a calcium oxalate stone.

2 Although salts of oxalic acid are white, these stones are brown or black. Their sharp surface traumatizes the uroepithelium and the colour is due to blood pigment.

3 Urinary frequency, dysuria and haematuria.

4 A plain X-ray of the pelvis almost invariably demonstrates the stone because of its high calcium content. Cystoscopy enables the stone to be visualized.

5 Calcium, ammonium and magnesium phosphate ('triple phosphate stone', see Question 113) and uric acid or urate stone.

(See Chapter 42, *Lecture Notes on General Surgery*.)

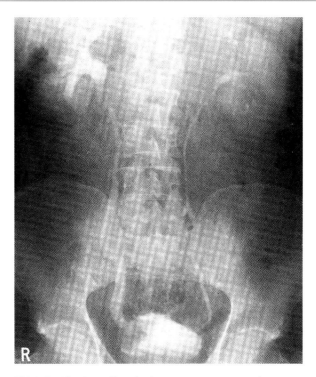

This is the 15-minute film of an intravenous urogram series on a man of 62, who presented with painless haematuria. Clinical examination was entirely negative.

1 Describe the abnormal findings in this film.

2 What is the radiological diagnosis?

3 What special investigation needs to be carried out in order to clinch the diagnosis?

4 What is the likely histological nature of this lesion?

5 What factors predispose to the development of bladder cancer?

1 There is an irregular filling defect in the right side of the bladder in the region of the ureteric orifice. There is dilatation of the right ureter.

2 A bladder tumour, which is obstructing the right ureter. The fact that the ureter is obstructed is in favour of a bladder cancer rather than a benign tumour.

3 Cystoscopy with transurethral biopsy.

4 Transitional cell carcinoma is by far the commonest bladder cancer.

5 There is a raised incidence of bladder cancer in smokers. There is a high incidence of malignant change in the exposed bladder mucosa of ectopia vesicae and in the bladder infested with schistosomiasis. Malignant change may also take place within a bladder diverticulum. Bladder tumours were extremely common among aniline dye and rubber workers because of the excretion of carcinogens (such as beta naphthylamine) in the urine.

(See Chapter 42, *Lecture Notes on General Surgery.*)

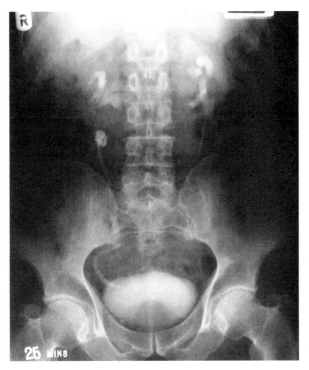

This is one of an intravenous urogram series taken of a patient aged 70 years, who presented with marked symptoms of prostatic obstruction.

1 What evidence can you see here of prostatic enlargement?

2 What are the appearances of the lower ends of the ureters?

3 What radiological evidence do you look for of bladder outlet obstruction?

4 Apart from the urinary tract, what else should you look for on an X-ray in such a case?

5 There are two other obvious abnormalities on this film—one of the kidneys, the other not related to the urinary tract. What are they?

1 Intravesical enlargement of the prostate is shown by a globular filling defect at the base of the bladder.

2 The terminations of the ureters are hooked upwards due to the enlarged prostate pushing up the trigone of the bladder.

3 There will be considerable post-micturition retention of urine in the bladder, the bladder wall will be thickened and may demonstrate diverticula. The urogram may show evidence of back pressure on the kidneys (hydronephrosis and hydroureter).

4 The films of the lumbar spine and bony pelvis should be scrutinized for evidence of secondary deposits, frequently sclerotic, which are present in about 25% of cases of carcinoma of the prostate.

5 The patient has horseshoe kidneys (note the way the renal pelvises point laterally). In addition, he has a calcified mesenteric lymph node, due to old tuberculous disease, on the right side.

(See Chapter 43, *Lecture Notes on General Surgery*.)

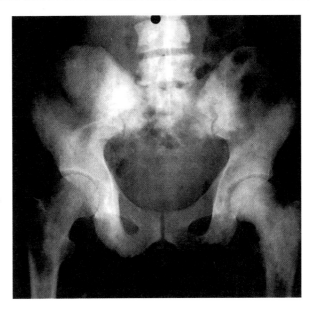

This is the X-ray of the pelvis of a patient aged 75, admitted with acute retention of urine.

1 What does the X-ray demonstrate?
2 Why are these appearances typical of prostatic carcinoma?
3 List the other tumours that commonly metastasize to bone.
4 What is a common emergency complication of a bony secondary?
5 How can prostatic bony secondaries be treated?

1 Multiple osteosclerotic secondaries.

2 Prostatic carcinoma typically produces osteosclerotic secondaries, whereas other secondary deposits are commonly osteoporotic.

3 Carcinomas of the lung, breast, kidney and thyroid typically metastasize to bone. These primary tumours, together with carcinoma of the prostate, account for the source of the vast majority of bony secondary deposits.

4 A pathological fracture.

5 Stilboestrol 1 mg three times a day or other techniques of hormonal manipulation may be employed. Local pain may be relieved by radiotherapy.

(See Chapter 43, *Lecture Notes on General Surgery*.)

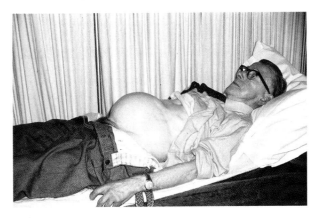

This elderly man, after a long period of increasing difficulty with micturition, has finally become totally unable to empty his bladder. Rectal examination revealed a very enlarged, but benign-feeling, prostate.

1 What does abdominal inspection reveal?

2 What physical sign will confirm that this swelling is the urinary bladder?

3 What are the possible causes of retention of urine without there being an obstruction to the urethra?

4 Apart from benign prostatic hypertrophy, what other local causes are there for retention of urine?

5 What would be the clinical features that would suggest uraemia in a patient such as this?

1 The bladder is enormously distended.

2 The percussion note over the suprapubic swelling is entirely dull.

3 The general causes of retention of urine can be classified into:

(a) Post-operative.

(b) CNS disease, e.g. multiple sclerosis, spinal compression from tumour, etc.

(c) Drugs, e.g. Pro-banthine.

4 Other local causes can be classified into:

(a) Within the lumen of the urethra — stone or blood clot.

(b) In the urethral wall — stricture.

(c) Outside the wall — malignant prostatic enlargement or occasionally pressure from faecal impaction or from a pelvic tumour.

5 The patient with uraemia may complain of headache, anorexia and vomiting. He may be drowsy and have a dry coated tongue.

(See Chapter 43, *Lecture Notes on General Surgery*.)

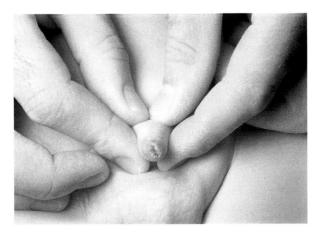

The parents brought this boy, aged 3 years, to the out-patient clinic because his foreskin would not retract. They noticed that his prepuce ballooned during micturition.

1 What is the diagnosis?

2 What often leads to the development of this condition?

3 What is the natural history of the prepuce in children?

4 What is the function of the prepuce in babies?

5 List your indications for advising circumcision in children.

1 Phimosis — this term implies gross narrowing of the preputial orifice.

2 Although this may occur as a congenital lesion, it usually results from the trauma of attempts at forcible retraction of the prepuce or as a result of chronic balanitis.

3 The prepuce is normally non-retractile in the first few months of life, due to congenital adhesions between the glans and prepuce. By the end of the first year 50% retract, and the vast majority can be retracted by the third or fourth year.

4 The prepuce protects the glans and urethral orifice from the excoriation of ammoniacal dermatitis.

5 Circumcision may be carried out in children for religious grounds, when organic phimosis is present (as in the present case) or in those instances where the prepuce cannot be retracted after the age of 4.

(See Chapter 45, *Lecture Notes on General Surgery*.)

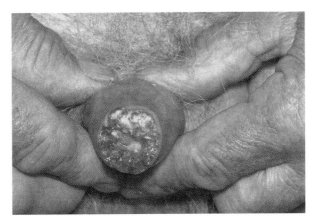

This elderly patient presented with a foul-smelling and ulcerated lesion of the penis.

1 What will be the likely histological diagnosis?
2 How does this tumour spread?
3 What group of men are immune from this disease?
4 What is the usual cause of death?
5 How is this type of tumour treated?

1 Squamous carcinoma of the penis.

2 (a) *Local*: the tumour may fungate through the prepuce and may spread along the shaft of the penis to destroy its substance.

(b) *Lymphatic*: to the inguinal lymph nodes.

(c) *Blood-borne*: spread to the lungs occurs late and is unusual.

3 It is virtually unknown among Jews, who are circumcised soon after birth.

4 Haemorrhage from fungating inguinal lymph nodes.

5 If the urethra is intact, treatment is by radiotherapy. If the urethra is involved, amputation of the penis. If the lymph nodes are involved and are operable, block dissection is performed, otherwise radiotherapy is given to the nodes if these are matted together and fixed.

(See Chapter 45, *Lecture Notes on General Surgery*.)

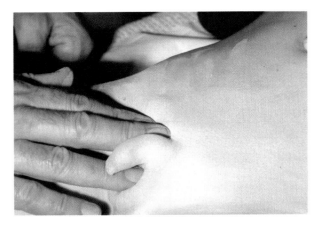

This 7-year-old boy has a normally placed left testicle. The right scrotum is empty but there is an obvious bulge in the right groin, which can be seen above the examiner's index finger. This testis cannot be coaxed into the scrotum.

1 What is the diagnosis?

2 What is meant by the term 'retractile testis'?

3 Where exactly is the right testis lying in this case, and how do you know it is not within the inguinal canal?

4 What are the complications of this condition?

5 What treatment should be advised for this patient?

1 Ectopic testicle.

2 Retractile testis is a normal testicle where an excessively active cremasteric reflex draws the testis up to the external inguinal ring. On careful examination it can be coaxed into the scrotum.

3 The testis is easily visible and is therefore lying in the superficial inguinal pouch, having emerged from the external ring. If it were still lying within the inguinal canal it would certainly not be visible and would probably not even be palpable.

4 Complications of this condition are:

    (a) Defective spermatogenesis — sterility if bilateral.

    (b) Increased risk of torsion.

    (c) Increased risk of trauma.

    (d) Increased risk of malignant change, which appears to be true even if surgical correction is carried out.

5 Orchidopexy (mobilization and placement of the testis into the scrotum) should be carried out as early as possible. The co-existing inguinal hernial sac should be removed at the same time.

(See Chapter 46, *Lecture Notes on General Surgery*.)

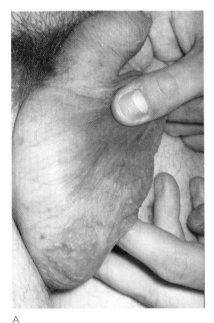

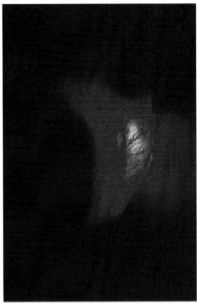

A   B

These photographs are of a patient aged 45. A smooth mass was felt in the right scrotum above and separate from a normal-sized testis.

1 What is the diagnosis?

2 What does (B) demonstrate?

3 What may be the appearance of the contents of this cyst?

4 Can these cysts be multiple and/or bilateral?

5 What treatment would you advise?

1 Cyst of the epididymis.

2 The cyst brilliantly transilluminates, whereas the adjacent testis does not do so.

3 The fluid may be water-clear or may be milky and contain sperm.

4 Cysts of the epididymis are not infrequently multiple and may be bilateral.

5 A small cyst that does not worry the patient can be left alone. Large cysts, which may be uncomfortable, should be removed surgically.

(See Chapter 46, *Lecture Notes on General Surgery*.)

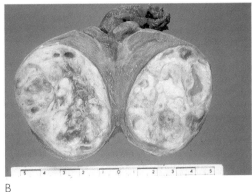

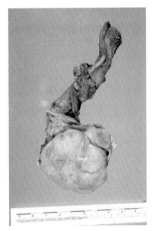

A

B

These photographs show the cut surface of two testes, which were removed surgically. (A) is from a man aged 37 years, (B) is from a 17-year-old.

1 What is the diagnosis of (A) and what is its histological appearance?

2 What is the diagnosis of (B) and what may be seen under the microscope?

3 What are the likely physical signs in the examination of the testis in cases such as these?

4 Describe the pathway of lymphatic spread of these tumours.

5 What is their blood-borne spread?

1 Seminoma. Sheets of cells, which vary from well-differentiated spermatocytes to undifferentiated round cells.

2 Teratoma. Microscopically the cells are very variable and the tumour may contain cartilage, bone, muscle, fat and other tissues. The rare variety of chorionephithelioma consists of syncytial tissue.

3 The testis usually presents as a painless hard mass, frequently associated with an overlying secondary hydrocele, which may contain blood-stained, rather than clear, yellow fluid.

4 Lymphatic spread is to the para-aortic nodes via the lymphatics, which accompany the testicular vein. Spread may then occur along the thoracic duct to the supraclavicular nodes, especially on the left side.

5 Blood-borne spread occurs to the lungs and liver. This is relatively early in teratoma and tends to be late in seminoma.

(See Chapter 46, *Lecture Notes on General Surgery*.)

CASES

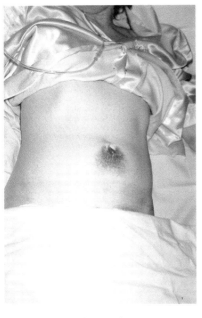 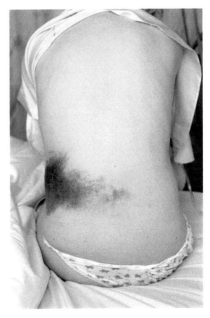

1 What are these two eponymous signs?
2 What is the mechanism of the appearance of the signs?
3 With what conditions are they associated?

1 Cullen's* and Grey Turner's† signs.

2 They are due to extravasation of blood, which tracks extraperitoneally round to the flank and through the umbilical cicatrix.

3 They are associated with causes of retroperitoneal haemorrhage, such as acute haemorrhagic pancreatitis, ruptured abdominal aortic or iliac aneurysm, and ruptured ectopic pregnancy.

(See Chapter 32, *Lecture Notes on General Surgery.*)

---

* Thomas Cullen (1868–1953), a gynaecologist at Johns Hopkins, Baltimore, USA, described peri-umbilical bluish discoloration in a case of ruptured ectopic pregnancy in 1922.

† George Grey Turner (1877–1951), a surgeon from Newcastle upon Tyne and later the Royal Postgraduate Medical School, Hammersmith Hospital, London, described this as a feature of acute pancreatitis in 1920.

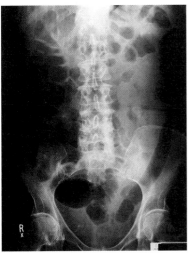

A

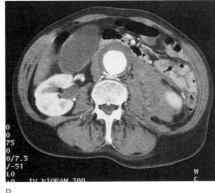

B

These are the X-rays of Case 1. She was a 72-year-old woman who presented with a 2-hour history of severe abdominal pain of sudden onset, radiating into her upper lumbar spine. With the onset of the pain she fainted.

1 What do these investigations show?

2 What complication has occurred?

3 What other complications can occur with the underlying condition?

4 What criteria are used to judge the timing of the elective treatment of the condition?

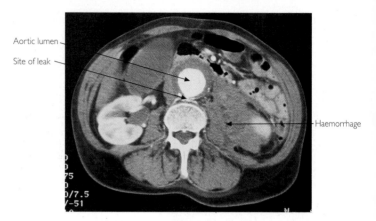

Aortic lumen
Site of leak
Haemorrhage

1 (A) is an abdominal X-ray and shows an absence of the left psoas shadow and the descending colon moved laterally with the appearance of being stretched around something medially. (B) is a CT scan and shows a 6 cm abdominal aortic aneurysm with a rind of thrombus (called mural thrombus) around the lumen, which is white due to the administration of contrast medium. The rind is deficient posteriorly, the site of a rupture. There is extensive haemorrhage around the lower pole of the left kidney, and the descending colon is seen stretched postero-laterally around the haematoma.

2 Rupture of an abdominal aotic aneurysm.

3 Aneurysms may rupture, erode into adjacent structures producing fistulas, such as aorto-caval and aorto-enteric fistulas; thrombosis and distal embolism of the contents of the sac may also occur. This woman had a successful operation.

4 Elective aneurysms are repaired when the risk of death from elective surgery is outweighed by the annual risk of rupture. Pain and tenderness are indications of more urgent repair, as are thrombosis and distal embolism. Assuming the patient is otherwise well, with no increased cardiac risk factors, an abdominal aortic aneurysm is repaired once it is in excess of 5.5 cm in anteroposterior diameter, measured by ultrasound scan.

(See Chapter 10, *Lecture Notes on General Surgery.*)

ant.parallel-5mins

pinhole-15mins

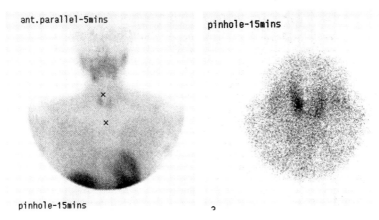

pinhole-15mins

A 33-year-old woman presented with a history of malaise, abdominal pain and constipation. Six months previously she had undergone surgery for a perforated peptic ulcer. Investigations showed a corrected calcium of 2.71 mmol/l (normal range 2.20–2.60), and a parathyroid hormone level of 69 (normal range 9–54). The results of the scan are shown above.

1 What is the diagnosis based on the blood tests?
2 What is the investigation and what does it show?
3 What treatment would you perform?
4 What other diagnoses should be considered from the history?

259

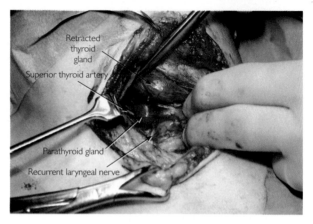

Retracted thyroid gland

Superior thyroid artery

Parathyroid gland

Recurrent laryngeal nerve

1 The patient has a raised serum calcium and a raised parathyroid hormone level, indicating hyperparathyroidism. The symptoms of abdominal pain and constipation are typical.

2 This is a Sestamibi scan, used to locate parathyroid adenomas; one can be seen on the right side of the neck in the inferior position.

3 The treatment of choice is a parathyroidectomy. The figure above illustrates the procedure, with the abnormal gland demonstrated behind the lower pole of the thyroid.

4 Parathyroid tumours may occur spontaneously, but may also be part of a multiple endocrine neoplasia (MEN) syndrome. The history of a previous peptic ulcer may be attributed to a gastrin-secreting tumour of the pancreas, and gastrin levels should be measured. This was not the case in this woman.

(See Chapter 38, *Lecture Notes on General Surgery.*)

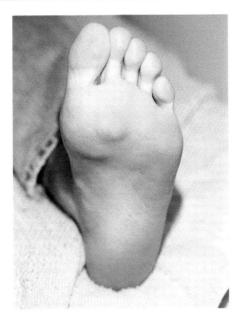

A 40-year-old carpenter presented with a 3-month history of this lump on the sole of his foot, which had been enlarging over that time. On direct questioning he recalled treading on a nail, which entered his foot at or near that site 6 months previously.

1 What is the likely diagnosis?

2 Lesions such as this may be classified into two forms, congenital and acquired. What is the other commonly used classification?

3 Where are such lesions more commonly found?

1 This is a dermoid cyst.

2 Dermoid cysts are alternatively classified as implantation and sequestration dermoids. This is an implantation dermoid.

3 Implantation dermoids are commonly found on the hand, often in gardeners as a result of rose thorn injuries. Sequestration dermoids are found at the sites of fusion of embryological plates, such as around the eye (external and internal angular dermoid).

(See Chapter 7, *Lecture Notes on General Surgery.*)

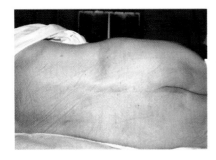
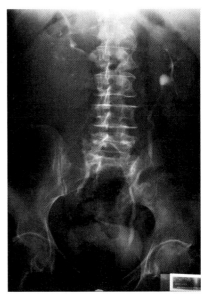

A 64-year-old woman presented with a painful swelling in her right loin, associated with a pyrexia of 38.5°C. Blood cultures were positive for *Staphylococcus aureus*. The clinical photograph shows her lying left side down.

1 What abnormality is visible on the clinical photograph?
2 What is the investigation on the right and what does it show?
3 What is the diagnosis and what is the treatment?

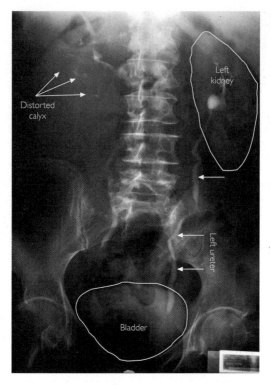

1 There is an area of erythema overlying a swelling in the right flank.

2 This is an intravenous urogram (IVU), in which an intravenous injection of contrast material has been given, and its excretion by the kidneys observed as it outlines the kidneys, ureters and bladder. This IVU shows contrast in the left renal pelvis and ureter with some also collecting in the bladder. However, the right kidney is abnormal, with a distorted renal pelvis, which appears to be leaking contrast.

3 This woman has a perinephric abscess, which requires open drainage. The distortion of the loin with overlying erythema is clearly visible on the clinical picture. The source of the infection was rupture of a renal carbuncle into the perinephric space, the carbuncle itself being caused by haematogenous seeding of the renal cortex with *Staphylococcus aureus*.

(See Chapter 41, *Lecture Notes on General Surgery*.)

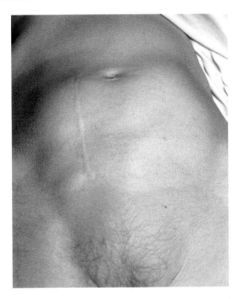

This 56-year-old woman presented with a 1-day history of vomiting and colicky central abdominal pain. She had felt 'bloated' for 2 days previously. Her bowel habit was irregular, and she last opened her bowels on the day before admission.

1 What can you see on inspection?
2 What is the diagnosis, and what is the likely cause?
3 How can you classify the causes of this appearance?
4 What factors will dictate your management in this case?

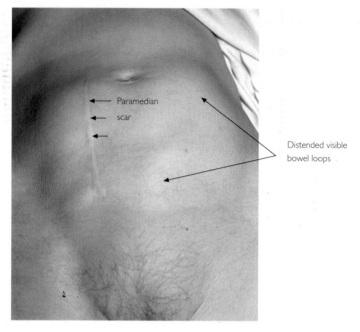

Paramedian scar

Distended visible bowel loops

I This is a photograph of the abdomen. There is a paramedian scar in the right iliac fossa (used for an appendicectomy when she was younger) and the abdomen itself is distended, with visibly distended bowel loops.

2 The diagnosis is intestinal obstruction. The fact that vomiting occurred before absolute constipation suggests a high (small bowel) obstruction. Since the patient has had previous surgery, the most likely diagnosis would be adhesive obstruction.

3 The causes of intestinal obstruction can be classified according to whether they are within the lumen (e.g. a bolus of food, a gallstone or faeces), in the wall (e.g. a tumour), or outside the wall (e.g. adhesions, the boundaries of a hernia sac).

4 The first thing to decide is whether there is any evidence of strangulation (tachycardia, pyrexia, colicky pain becoming constant, leucocytosis). If so, a laparotomy is indicated to divide the adhesions. Other indications for laparotomy include unresolving obstruction in spite of treatment, and the presence of a mass. Otherwise treatment is intravenous fluid replacement and nasogastric aspiration.

(See Chapter 21, *Lecture Notes on General Surgery*.)

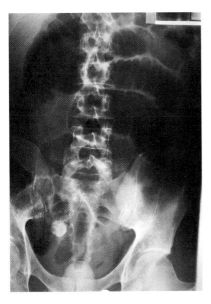
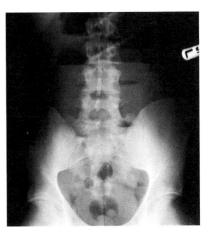

These X-rays are of a 22-year-old PhD student, who presented with a 5-day history of colicky central abdominal pain, and vomiting for the last 2 days. On direct questioning he complained of feeling distended. On examination he was pyrexial (37.9°C) and was tender in the right iliac fossa. He had a leucocytosis of 20.5×10^9/l. He had never been to hospital before.

I Describe the X-ray appearances.

2 There are two diagnoses here, one causing the other. What are the diagnoses?

3 What management plan would you institute?

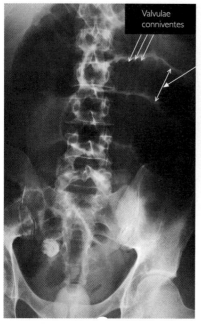

Valvulae conniventes

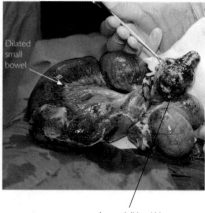

Dilated small bowel

Appendolith within a very distended appendix

1 The X-ray shows multiple dilated loops of bowel. The loops are centrally placed and there are band markings across the whole diameter (valvulae conniventes), signifying dilated small bowel. The X-ray on the right is an erect X-ray demonstrating multiple fluid levels.

2 The diagnosis is small bowel obstruction. There is a radio-opaque circular lesion in the pelvis on the right, which may be related to the cause. The patient's age would be against a diagnosis of gall stone ileus, as would be the absence of air in the biliary tree on either film. In fact this is a large stone (appendolith) within a distended and inflamed appendix, to which is stuck small bowel (an appendix mass).

3 The patient has not had any previous surgery and is toxic (tachycardia and pyrexial). He therefore merits a laparotomy to determine the cause of obstruction. Before any operation he should be fully resuscitated with intravenous fluids, and a nasogastric tube passed to decompress his distended small intestine and reduce the risk of aspiration on induction of anaesthesia.

(See Chapters 21 and 24, *Lecture Notes on General Surgery*.)

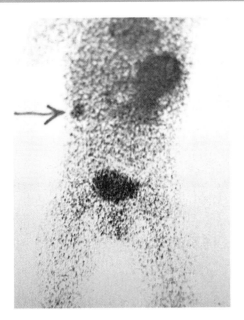

A 7-year-old boy presented with a day's history of rectal bleeding, passing dark red blood and clots. On examination there is no palpable mass. The above radionuclide scan was performed using technetium.

1 What does the scan show?
2 What is the diagnosis?
3 What is the treatment?

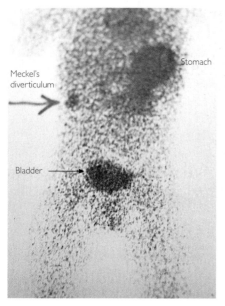

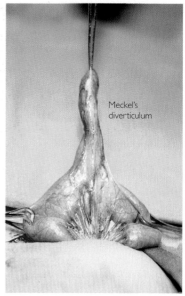

1 The scan is a radionuclide technetium scan, which shows uptake in the region of the bladder and stomach. In addition there is an area of uptake arrowed on the right side. The radionuclide is taken up by gastric parietal cells in both the stomach, and also in any ectopic mucosa in a Meckel's diverticulum.* Apparent uptake in the bladder is due to its excretion in urine.

2 The boy is bleeding from a peptic ulcer in the adjacent normal ileum secondary to the acid which is being produced by the parietal cell mucosa within the Meckel's diverticulum.

3 The boy should be resuscitated, transfused as necessary, and undergo urgent laparotomy to remove the Meckel's diverticulum.

(See Chapters 20 and 23, *Lecture Notes on General Surgery.*)

---

* Johann Frederick Meckel (1781–1833): Professor of Anatomy and Surgery, Halle, Germany.

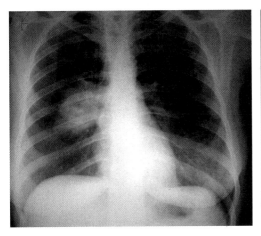 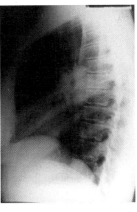

A 45-year-old woman presented with a 6-month history of a dry cough, and more recently occasional episodes of haemoptysis. On direct questioning she complained of pain in her wrists and ankles. The postero-anterior (PA) and lateral chest X-rays are shown above.

1 What is the principal abnormality on the X-ray?
2 What is the likely cause of the abnormality?
3 What is the likely cause of the wrist and ankle pains?
4 How would you manage this patient?

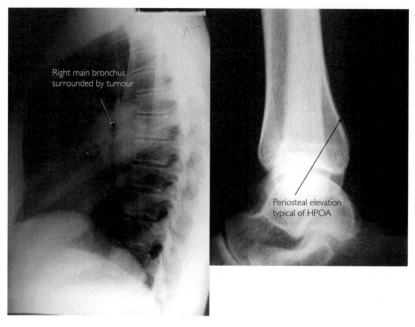

Right main bronchus
surrounded by tumour

Periosteal elevation
typical of HPOA

1 There is an opacity adjacent to the right cardiac silhouette on the PA film, which is shown to surround the right bronchus on the lateral film.

2 This is a bronchial carcinoma.

3 In the context of a bronchial carcinoma, the pains may be due to hyper-trophic pulmonary osteoarthropathy (HPOA). This is confirmed on the X-ray above, which shows the periosteal reaction. The patient also had finger clubbing, which is often associated with HPOA.

4 The first priority of management is to confirm the diagnosis. With such a proximal tumour this is best done by flexible bronchoscopy and biopsy, which in this case revealed a squamous carcinoma. Having confirmed this, the next step is to see whether it is resectable. For this one needs to be sure that there is no spread of the carcinoma, and this is assessed by computed tomography (CT) of chest and abdomen, with biopsy of any suspiciously enlarged nodes. In the absence of disease elsewhere, resection of the carcinoma can be performed, assuming that the patient's respiratory reserve is sufficient. In this case the patient underwent a pneumonectomy.

(See Chapter 8, *Lecture Notes on General Surgery.*)

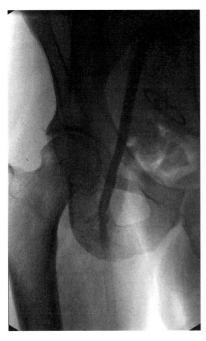
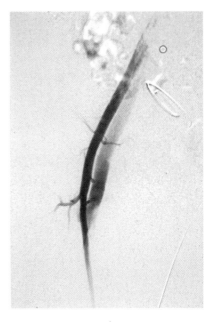

A 45-year-old man with chronic renal failure developed a painful swelling in his right groin 6 weeks after having a large cannula inserted in the right femoral vein for acute haemodialysis, prior to having a peritoneal dialysis catheter inserted. He had also noticed progressive claudication in the right leg over the same period of time. On examination he had a small lump in the groin with a palpable thrill. On auscultation there was a loud bruit. An angiogram (above) was performed, with a catheter passed through the left femoral artery.

1 What does the angiogram show?
2 How can you explain such findings?
3 What is the explanation of the new onset claudication?
4 How would you manage this complication?
5 What is the difference between the above pathology and a false aneurysm of the femoral artery?

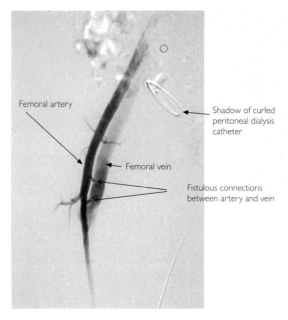

Femoral artery

Shadow of curled peritoneal dialysis catheter

Femoral vein

Fistulous connections between artery and vein

1 The angiogram shows contrast in the femoral artery, with early filling of the femoral vein due to two connections, fistulae, between the femoral artery and femoral vein. The image on the left on the previous page is a conventional X-ray, while the image on the right is created by digitally subtracting a control image from a subsequent image, after contrast medium has been administered. This is known as digital subtraction imaging.

2 At the time of insertion of the haemodialysis catheter it passed through the artery into the vein. Such was the difficulty with the placement of the catheter that several attempts were made before a successful venepuncture was achieved, accounting for the multiple fistulae.

3 The claudication is accounted for by the shunting of arterial blood across the fistulae, resulting in reduced perfusion of the distal vessels, and claudication on exercise.

4 The fistulae should be closed, since they are already causing symptoms and will enlarge over time, placing the limb in jeopardy. The fistulous tracks could be embolized at angiography or, as in this case, explored surgically and closed formally.

5 A false aneurysm occurs when an artery is damaged and blood leaks into the surrounding tissues, which contain the blood. A surrounding rim of thrombus forms. There is no connection with the adjacent vein.

(See Chapter 10, *Lecture Notes on General Surgery*.)

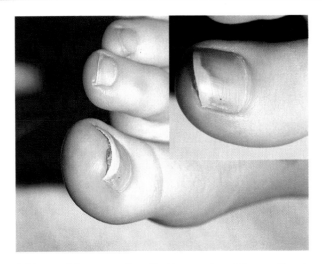

A 16-year-old boy was referred by his general practitioner with an ingrowing toe nail. A full history revealed that the boy's main symptom was a sensation of pressure in the toe, and pain when it was knocked.

1 Describe the abnormality in the photograph. Do you think this is an ingrowing toe nail?

2 What is the likely diagnosis and how would you prove it?

3 What is the management of this condition?

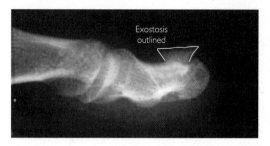

1 The nail margins are not inflamed and the nail itself is lifted from the nail bed at its tip, with the suggestion, on close examination, of something pushing it up. This is not an ingrowing toe nail.

2 The most likely diagnosis is a subungual exostosis, which can be demonstrated on a lateral X-ray of the hallux (above).

3 The condition is managed by initial avulsion of the nail to reveal the underlying exostosis, which is then excised from the distal phalanx of the hallux. The nail should grow back normally since the germinal matrix is seldom involved.

(See Chapter 7, *Lecture Notes on General Surgery*.)

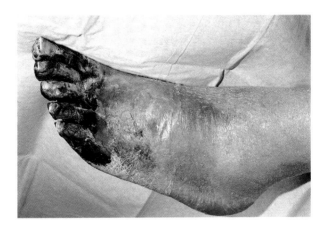

This is the foot of a 65-year-old diabetic.

1 Describe the features.

2 What is the likely cause?

3 What treatment would you recommend?

4 In broad terms, what are the three indications for amputation of a limb?

1 The toes and distal foot are black and mummified, typical of dry gangrene. There is oedema of the ankle. The skin over the ankle is pink and healthy, although there is a dark area over the dorsal proximal foot, which may represent ischaemia.

2 The foot has become gangrenous due to ischaemia. This is due to arterial disease, and in a diabetic with this pattern of limb loss, small vessel disease is likely to be the predominant factor.

3 In the absence of any correctable vascular lesion the limb may be left either to demarcate and be debrided, or a formal proximal amputation may be performed — in this case a below-knee amputation.

4 A convenient classification of the indications for amputation is that a limb is dead (e.g. ischaemia), dangerous (e.g. osteosarcoma, gas gangrene) or useless (e.g. following extensive trauma).

(See Chapter 10, *Lecture Notes on General Surgery*.)

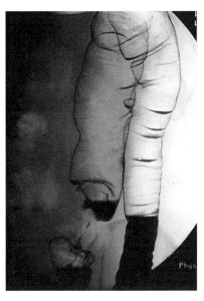 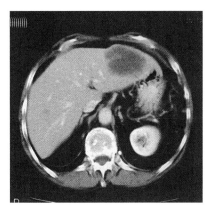

A 64-year-old man presented with an 8-month history of change in bowel habit. A double contrast barium enema (left) was performed.

1 What is the principle abnormality and what is the likely diagnosis?

2 Following surgery to the primary lesion he was followed up in the clinic, and a CT scan 6 months later revealed the abnormality above (right). What does the CT scan show and what is the likely diagnosis?

3 How would you manage this patient?

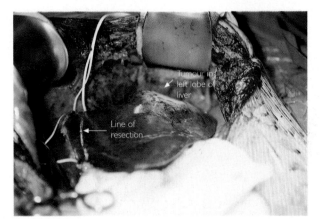

1 There is a stricture in the distal transverse colon typical of a carcinoma. The patient underwent a transverse colectomy, which confirmed an adenocarcinoma of the colon with spread through the wall, but without lymph node involvement: a Dukes' B carcinoma.

2 The CT scan shows a 5 cm diameter lesion in the left lobe of the liver typical of a secondary deposit from the previous colon carcinoma. There is a second small 1 cm lesion in the right lobe, which was found to be a haemangioma.

3 The patient needs a full radiological evaluation including a chest CT scan to determine whether there is any other site of tumour spread. Assuming that the patient is fit enough and there is no evidence of tumour elsewhere, the patient should be considered for a left hemihepatectomy. The photograph above illustrates the operation at a point when the left hepatic artery is ligated and the surface has been marked along the line of resection.

(See Chapters 25 and 30, *Lecture Notes on General Surgery.*)

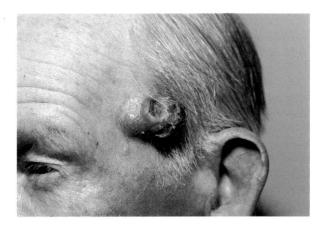

A 71-year-old man attended his general practitioner 2 years previously with a presumed sebaceous cyst on his temple, which was removed in the surgery. He now presents with an ulcerating lump at the site of the previous excision.

1 Describe the lesion.

2 What other area would you like to examine, if any?

3 How would you investigate this lesion?

4 What is the differential diagnosis?

1 There is a 2 × 1cm raised lesion on the left temple just above, and anterior to, the ear. The surface is ulcerated in more than one area and the ulcer edges appear rolled.

2 This may be a malignant lesion, so it is important to palpate the regional lymph nodes for evidence of regional spread. This will influence subsequent management, and the presence of hard nodes may affect your diagnosis of the primary lesion.

3 The lesion should be biopsied to determine its nature. This is best performed as an excision biopsy.

4 With a history of a previously excised sebaceous cyst it is possible that this is an example of Cock's peculiar tumour.* However, the rolled ulcerated edges are more in keeping with the real diagnosis, a squamous cell carcinoma.

(See Chapter 7, *Lecture Notes on General Surgery*.)

---

* Edward Cock (1805–1892): Surgeon, Guy's Hospital, London.

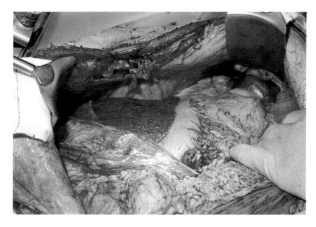

This is an operative photograph of a patient with primary sclerosing cholangitis.

1 What signs of portal hypertension are visible at surgery?

2 Where would you expect to find varices in patients with portal hypertension?

3 What options exist other than liver transplantation for reducing portal hypertension?

4 What more common conditions are associated with primary sclerosing cholangitis?

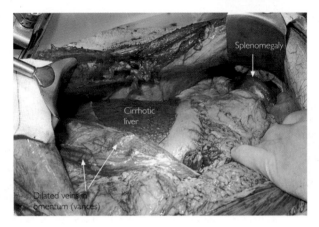

1 As illustrated above, the liver is cirrhotic. There are dilated veins (varices) in the omentum and the tip of an enlarged spleen can also be seen in the left upper quadrant.

2 Varices normally occur at sites where the portal circulation comes into contact with the systemic venous circulation. This includes along the oesophagogastric junction (oesophageal varices), along the umbilical vein, which may be recanalized resulting in a *caput medusa* around the umbilicus, along the inferior mesenteric vein to cause anorectal varices, and along the ligamentous attachments of the liver to the diaphragm and retroperitoneum.

3 Acutely portal hypertension may be reduced medically with vasopressin or octreotide infusions. Longer-term control may be helped by propranolol. Surgical options include spleno-renal and mesenteric–caval fistulae. However, surgical options have now been replaced by trans-internal jugular portosystemic shunt (TIPS).

4 Primary sclerosing cholangitis (PSC) is associated with inflammatory bowel disease such as ulcerative colitis and Crohn's disease.

(See Chapter 30, *Lecture Notes on General Surgery*.)

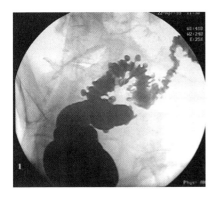 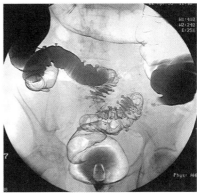

A 65-year-old man presented with a 3-month history of abdominal distension and colicky lower abdominal pain. For 2 days before admission he had not passed flatus or faeces, although this resolved shortly after admission.

1 What pathological process does the history suggest?

2 What abnormalities are visible on the barium enema above?

3 What is the pathological process in the bowel wall that causes the stricture seen on the barium enema?

4 Enumerate the complications of diverticular disease.

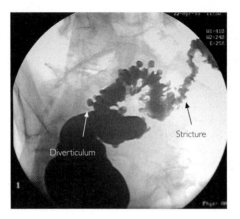

Stricture

Diverticulum

I The history is suggestive of large intestinal obstruction. The absence of vomiting is more suggestive of distal obstruction; early occurrence of vomiting before absolute constipation implies a higher intestinal obstruction.

2 The X-ray is a double contrast barium enema. The most obvious abnormality is a long stricture (highlighted above) in the sigmoid colon. There are multiple diverticula throughout the remaining bowel. This is a diverticular stricture. Ischaemic strictures are normally around the splenic flexure and malignant strictures tend to be much shorter and with rolled edges.

3 A diverticular stricture is due to muscular hypertrophy with no mucosal abnormality (see below).

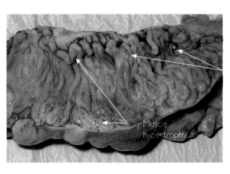

Faecal pellets
emerging from
diverticula

Muscle
hypertrophy

4 Diverticular disease usually presents with abdominal pain due to inflammation of a diverticulum (diverticulitis). Other complications include abscess formation, perforation, stricture, fistulation (particularly into the bladder, a colovesical fistula) and haemorrhage. Diverticular disease may co-exist with an adenocarcinoma of the colon, but there is no causal relationship.

(See Chapter 25, *Lecture Notes on General Surgery*.)

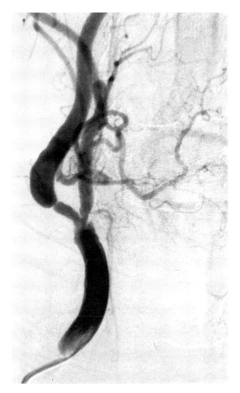

A 70-year-old man presented with a history that 4 weeks previously he had become blind in his right eye. The patient said the blindness came on as if someone was drawing a curtain down over his eye. The blindness lasted a few hours before he recovered. As part of the assessment this angiogram was taken of the right carotid artery.

1 What is the patient's presenting complaint usually called, and what does it mean?

2 What is the first-line special investigation for someone with this presentation?

3 When is angiography to be performed and what are its complications?

4 What does the angiogram show?

5 What treatment is indicated?

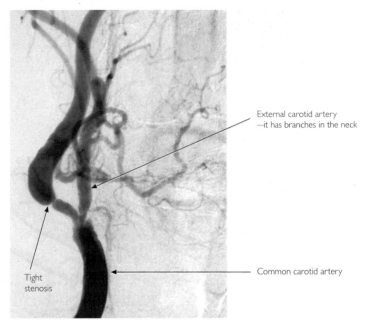

External carotid artery
—it has branches in the neck

Common carotid artery

Tight
stenosis

1 Amaurosis fugax, or fleeting blindness, due to embolism from the ipsilateral carotid artery.

2 Duplex of the carotid artery is usually done first because it is not invasive and can be readily performed with a good sensitivity for detecting a clinically significant stenosis (over 70% narrowing).

3 Angiography is performed when the duplex suggests complete occlusion, since this requires no treatment, whereas a tight stenosis does require treatment. The most important complication of angiography in this setting is distal embolization, resulting in strokes or transient ischaemia.

4 The angiogram shows a stenosis at the bifurcation of the carotid artery with a very tight stenosis in the internal carotid artery.

5 The stenosis is greater than 70%, therefore carotid endarterectomy is indicated to remove the diseased intima and reduce the chances of further embolization.

(See Chapter 10, *Lecture Notes on General Surgery*.)

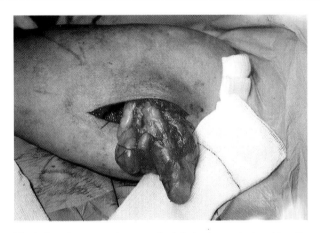

The lesion above was photographed during its surgical excision. It presented as a swelling on the patient's arm, which slowly increased in size over many years.

1 Describe the lesion. What is it?

2 What are the characteristics of the lesion on examination, and how would you differentiate it from a sebaceous cyst?

3 What complications may occur attributable to this lesion?

1 There is an incision in the skin out of which a yellow lobulated lesion has been partly removed. The lesion appears to have a defined capsule with small blood vessels stretched over its surface. The lesion is a lipoma.

2 A lipoma is a well-defined subcutaneous lesion that is soft and fluctuant. It is usually mobile, but may be in part within an underlying muscle and so appear tethered when that muscle contracts. A sebaceous cyst, in contrast, originates in sebaceous glands in the skin and as such is part of the skin—the skin cannot be moved over it. A punctum is usually visible on the surface of a sebaceous cyst, and absent over a lipoma.

3 Lipomas are benign tumours of adipose tissue and are usually of no clinical significance. Occasionally large lipomas may develop into liposarcomas, and a rapidly growing liposarcoma may be mistaken for a benign lipoma. In general a lipoma represents a source of worry for the patient, a source of mystery for the medical student, and a source of work for the surgeon.

(See Chapter 7, *Lecture Notes on General Surgery.*)

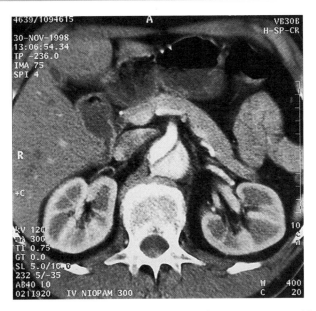

A 55-year-old hypertensive man presented as an emergency with a sudden severe pain in his chest, and later in his lumbar spine. He described the pain as tearing in nature. On examination his general practitioner noted he was shocked, hypertensive, and with no palpable pulses in either leg. On arrival at hospital he underwent an urgent CT scan (above).

1 From the clinical history what diagnoses should be considered?

2 What diagnosis is supported by the CT scan?

3 What factor influences the course of management?

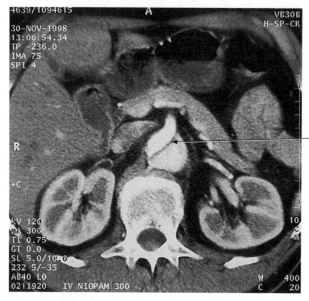

Septum dividing true lumen from false lumen

1 In any patient with severe chest pain the possibility of myocardial infarction should be considered. This patient had a history of a tearing pain rather than the crushing tight pain of a myocardial infarct. In addition the pain moved from the chest to the lumbar spine. This is highly suggestive of an aortic dissection.

2 The CT scan is at the level of the superior mesenteric artery. There is a septum across the aortic lumen typical of an aortic dissection. Contrast can be seen on either side of the septum.

3 Management of aortic dissection depends on the upper limit of the dissection. If this is in the ascending aorta or aortic arch (a Type A dissection) the patient requires surgery to interpose a piece of prosthetic aorta (usually made of Dacron). This prevents further retrograde dissection into the aortic root, in particular to stop dissection through a coronary cusp avulsing a coronary artery, or into the pericardium to cause an acute tamponade. A dissection that starts in the descending aorta (Type B) is managed by lowering the patient's blood pressure aggressively.

(See Chapter 9, *Lecture Notes on General Surgery.*)

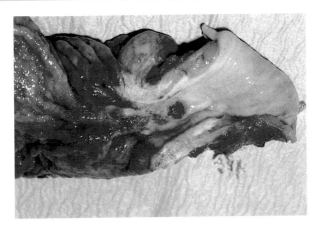

This is a surgical specimen from a 55-year-old man who presented with a 6-week history of dysphagia. At endoscopy he was found to have an ulcerating lesion at the oesophago-gastric junction. The lesion was biopsied and the ulcer found to be malignant. He underwent an oesophagogastrectomy.

1 What is the likely cell type of the malignant ulcer?

2 Describe the surgical specimen. What feature is particularly noteworthy of a cancer of the lower oesophagus?

3 What are the treatment options for such a tumour?

4 What investigations are usually performed prior to surgery on such a tumour? What is the prognosis?

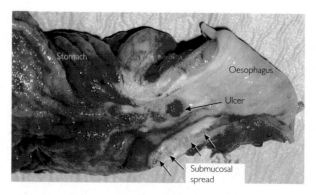

1 Lower third oesophageal tumours are usually adenocarcinoma; upper and middle third oesophageal tumours are squamous carcinoma.

2 This is a specimen including the lower third of the oesophagus and adjacent stomach. There is a 1 cm ulcer just above the oesophago-gastric junction. The ulcer has raised edges and a red inflamed base. The cut edge of the lower oesophagus shows a submucous infiltrate extending for a distance above and below the ulcer. This submucosal spread is typical of oesophageal tumours and in removing an oesophageal cancer the surgeon tries to remove at least 5 cm of oesophagus above the tumour to ensure microscopic clearance.

3 The tumour can be resected surgically or, if the growth is extensive and obliterating the lumen, a stent may be placed across it. Typical stents for oesophageal tumours are the Celestin and Nottingham tubes. Stents are placed at endoscopy. An alternative that is becoming more popular is laser vaporization of the tumour to create a lumen through the tumour. Radiotherapy has no place in adenocarcinoma, but may be useful in squamous carcinoma.

4 An endoscopic biopsy should be performed to confirm the diagnosis. The patient needs a CT scan of his chest and abdomen to exclude spread to the lymph nodes and adjacent structures. If a cure is not possible, palliation by stenting may be a preferred option. Lastly, the patient needs to be assessed from the anaesthetic point of view to see whether he is fit enough to withstand surgery.

(See Chapter 18, *Lecture Notes on General Surgery*.)

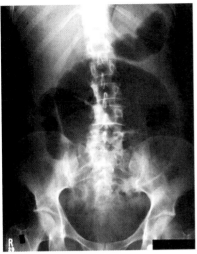 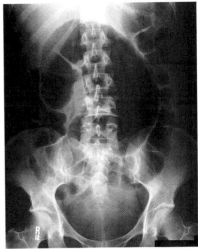

A 35-year-old woman presented with a 10-hour history of lower abdominal central colicky pain and distension. She had experienced similar episodes over the previous 2 years, which were thought to be due to 'irritable bowel syndrome'. The X-ray on the right was taken at presentation, the one on the left the following morning.

1 What do the X-rays show and what is the diagnosis?
2 How do you distinguish this condition from sigmoid volvulus?
3 What treatment is available?
4 What is the aetiology of the abnormality?

ن

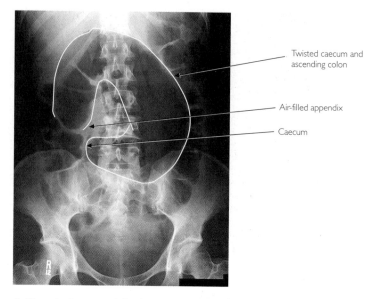

Twisted caecum and ascending colon

Air-filled appendix

Caecum

I There is a large centrally placed bowel loop with haustra crossing the diameter of the bowel. The loop forms an open C, with the opening towards the right iliac fossa. The caecum is not separately identified. Between the first and second film air passes into the distal colon. On the second film the air-filled appendix is just visible within the loop. This is the appearance of a partially obstructing caecal volvulus.

2 A sigmoid volvulus is often large and the axis is to the left iliac fossa rather than the right iliac fossa. In addition, in signal volvulus the caecum is usually visible in the right iliac fossa and may be dilated if the volvulus is long standing.

3 Because there is a tendency to intermittent volvulus and possible complete volvulus with strangulation, surgery is required. There are two surgical operations. One is to remove the offending caecum and perform a right hemicolectomy. This may be required in the face of ischaemia or infarction as a consequence of volvulus. Alternatively the caecum may be fixed to the right iliac fossa (caecopexy), either by caecostomy or by fashioning a fold or peritoneum.

4 The fundamental problem is a developmental one, akin to malrotation, except that in this instance the caecum has descended beyond its normal position. It has a narrow mesenteric pedicle around which it twists. Caecopexy will not correct this and is therefore an unsatisfactory procedure. Broadening the mesenteric pedicle, as is done in cases of malrotation, is a more appropriate procedure.

(See Chapter 22, *Lecture Notes on General Surgery.*)

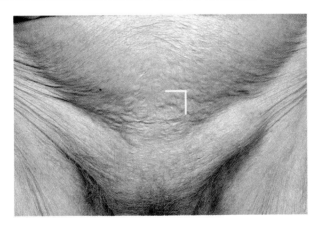

A 71-year-old woman presented with a lump in the left groin, which she had noticed 4 months previously.

1 What is the relationship of the lump to the pubic tubercle as marked on the photograph above?

2 What is the diagnosis?

3 What is the differential diagnosis of lumps in this site?

4 A Richter's hernia is common at this site. What is a Richter's hernia?

5 What treatment would you advise for the above lump?

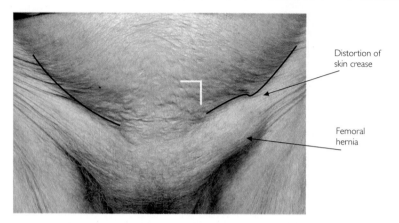

Distortion of skin crease

Femoral hernia

1 The lump is below and lateral to the pubic tubercle.

2 This is a left femoral hernia. Another feature is noted above, where the femoral hernia distorts the skin crease, unlike an inguinal hernia.

3 The differential diagnosis is best thought of by reference to the structures around the femoral canal as follows:

Femoral canal: femoral hernia

Femoral artery: aneurysm

Sapheno-femoral junction: saphena varix

Lymphatics: enlarged lymph node (called Cloquet's* node if in femoral canal)

Hip joint: synovial bursa

Subcutaneous fat: lipoma

Psoas sheath: psoas abscess

4 A Richter's[†] hernia is when only part of the wall of a loop of bowel is caught in a hernia sac. This produces incomplete obstruction and necrosis of the herniated bowel wall, which will go on to perforate.

5 Because of the risks of strangulation of a loop of bowel caught within, a femoral hernia should always be repaired.

(See Chapter 29, *Lecture Notes on General Surgery.*)

---

* Hippolyte Cloquet (1787–1840). Professor of Anatomy, Paris.
[†] August Richter (1742–1812). Surgeon, Göttingen, Germany.

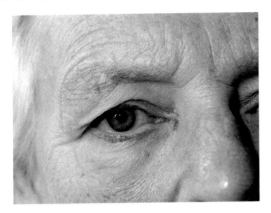

A 61-year-old woman presented with a lesion adjacent to the inner canthus of the right eye. On inspection the lesion has a raised pearly edge and a central ulcer.

1 What is the diagnosis?

2 Where else do these lesions occur?

3 What treatment would you advise?

4 What is the prognosis following complete excision?

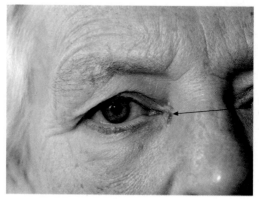

Basal cell
carcinoma

1 A basal cell carcinoma (rodent ulcer).

2 Basal cell carcinomas, like squamous cell carcinomas of the skin, arise in sun exposed areas of the body, particularly on the head above a line drawn from the angle of the mouth to the external auditary meatus, particularly around the inner canthus of the eye.

3 Surgical excision is usually recommended to avoid invasion of the lesion into adjacent structures. The tumours are radiosensitive so radiotherapy may be considered where surgery is not possible.

4 Basal cell carcinomas rarely metastasize, and following complete excision a complete cure is the rule.

(See Chapter 7, *Lecture Notes on General Surgery.*)

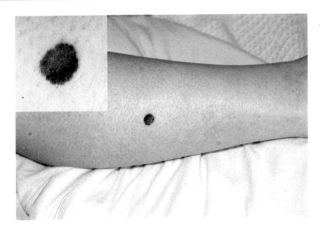

A 50-year-old woman has had a mole on her right leg since birth. Over the previous 6 years she has noticed the lump get slightly bigger and the colour darken.

1 Describe the lesion.

2 What is the most likely diagnosis?

3 How would you treat this lesion?

4 What is the likely prognosis of this lesion, and what is the most important factor?

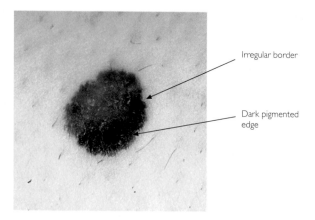

Irregular border

Dark pigmented edge

I There is a small I cm lesion on the anterior surface of the right leg. It is pigmented, the pigment being heterogeneous with a crescent of darker pigment on one side. The border is also irregular. There are no obvious satellite lesions and no evidence of bleeding.

2 This is a superficial spreading type of malignant melanoma.

3 The lesion should be excised with a good margin of clearance to obtain histological confirmation. Palpation of the regional lymph nodes in the right groin is necessary. Presence of palpable nodes would merit a block dissection in the absence of any further spread on imaging.

4 This is a flat lesion so the prognosis is good. The most important prognostic factor in melanoma is the thickness of the lesion. This was measured as 0.9 mm from top to bottom, a measure known as the Breslow thickness. This measure has replaced measurement relative to the skin layers as described by Clark (this lesion is Clark's level 3). Histology confirmed wide excision and absence of vascular invasion.

The 5-year survival following excision of a lesion of thickness up to 0.75 mm is over 95%, and with a lesion between 0.75 and 1.5 mm, as in this case, is 90%.

(See Chapter 7, *Lecture Notes on General Surgery.*)

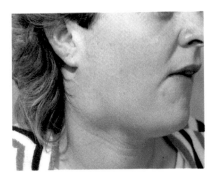
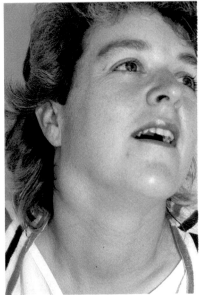

This 45-year-old woman noticed a swelling on the right side of her neck, which appeared just after she had had an upper respiratory tract infection.

1 What is the lesion?
2 From what is it derived?
3 What are the consequences of incomplete excision?
4 Between what two important structures in the neck may this arise?

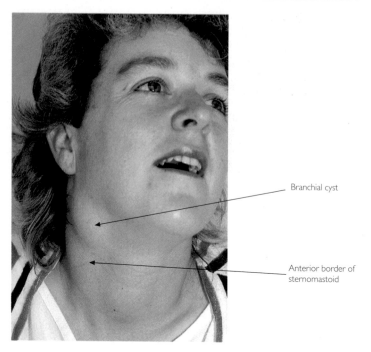

Branchial cyst

Anterior border of
sternomastoid

1 A branchial cyst. These lesions commonly get bigger following an upper respiratory tract infection.

2 A branchial cyst is traditionally thought to arise from remnants of the second branchial arch.

3 Incomplete excision may result in sinus formation at the site of excision.

4 A branchial cyst may have a connection that passes between the external and internal carotid arteries to the tonsillar fossa.

(See Chapter 36, *Lecture Notes on General Surgery.*)

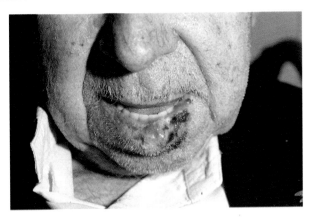

This 88-year-old man developed a non-healing ulcer on his lower lip, which has slowly enlarged over the previous 3 months.

1   What is the likely diagnosis?
2   What cell type is the lesion likely to be?
3   What particular features should be sought on examination?
4   What treatment can be offered?

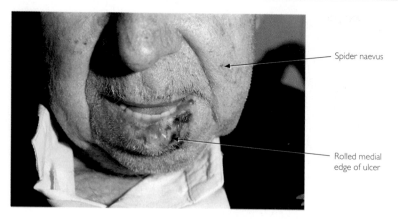

Spider naevus

Rolled medial
edge of ulcer

1 There is an ulcerating lesion on the left side of the lower lip. It has slightly raised edges and there is evidence of recent bleeding around its margins. The appearance, its position on the lower lip rather than the upper lip, and the history of slow growth are highly suggestive of a carcinoma.

2 Malignant lesions of the lip, like the majority of malignant diseases of the mouth and pharynx, are generally squamous carcinomas.

3 Examination should include assessment of the draining lymph nodes for spread, and also a thorough examination of the oral cavity for a synchronous tumour elsewhere.

4 Squamous carcinomas of the lip are usually excised. In this man's case, because of the protrusion of the lower lip, excision and primary closure was easily achieved. There were no pathological lymph nodes and no other lesions in the oral cavity.

(See Chapter 16, *Lecture Notes on General Surgery.*)

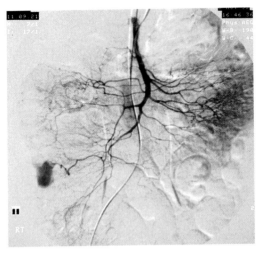

A 74-year-old man presented as an emergency with a history of passing blood and clots *per rectum*. The bleeding was described as filling half the pan. By the time he arrived in hospital the bleeding had subsided and no abnormality was detected on abdominal examination. Rectal examination revealed old blood, and sigmoidoscopy revealed blood-stained mucosa but no source of bleeding. His admission haemoglobin concentration was 13.5 g/dl. The following day his haemoglobin came back at 11.5 g/dl. At lunchtime the next day he had a further brisk bleed and had the above investigation performed.

1 Why did his haemoglobin fall 2 g/dl following admission, even though he had no further bleeds between samples?

2 What common causes of bleeding would you consider?

3 What is the examination above and what does it show?

4 How would you manage this patient?

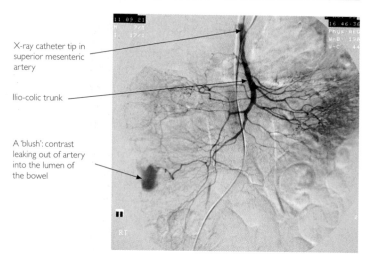

X-ray catheter tip in superior mesenteric artery

Ilio-colic trunk

A 'blush': contrast leaking out of artery into the lumen of the bowel

1 Following the bleed he was resuscitated with fluids but not blood. His circulating volume was replenished, causing a haemodilution. The fall signifies a blood loss of 2 g/dl, around 1 litre of blood.

2 Passage of fresh blood and clots suggests bleeding from the colon, although a briskly bleeding duodenal ulcer may rarely present this way. The commonest colonic cause in a man of his age would be diverticular disease, followed by a vascular malformation and a carcinoma.

3 The X-ray is a selective superior mesenteric arteriogram. Contrast is seen throughout the arterial tree and a pronounced blush is seen in the right iliac fossa, representing contrast and blood entering the ascending colon near the caecum. An arteriogram only detects bleeding when it is brisk and taking place at the time of arteriography, as was the case here.

4 The patient is actively bleeding. He needs an urgent laparotomy and, based on the localization of the bleeding by angiography, a right hemicolectomy should be performed. At surgery this patient was found to be bleeding from a diverticulum in the ascending colon, which had eroded into an adjacent vessel.

(See Chapter 25, *Lecture Notes on General Surgery.*)

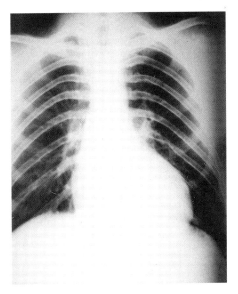

A 20-year-old medical student discovered he had hypertension while practising with a sphygmomanometer for the first time. His blood pressure was 180/110 mmHg when taken in his right arm while sitting at rest. A fellow medical student made the diagnosis of the cause of his raised blood pressure by palpating radial and femoral pulses simultaneously. During his assessment for surgery the above chest X-ray was taken.

1 What is the diagnosis, and what were the findings on palpating his pulses?
2 What features on the chest X-ray confirm the diagnosis?
3 Where is the problem and what is the treatment?
4 What is the principal risk of such surgery?

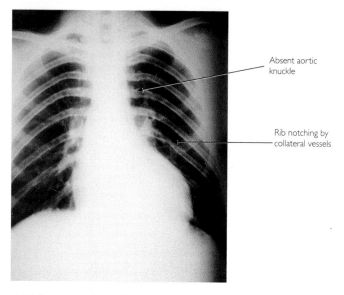

Absent aortic knuckle

Rib notching by collateral vessels

1 He has coarctation of the aorta. On palpation his femoral pulses were weak, and there was a delay in the pulse wave reaching the femoral artery compared to the radial pulse.

2 The chest X-ray shows absence of the aortic knuckle and rib notching due to the large collateral vessels taking blood distally.

3 The coarctation is usually just distal to the origin of the left subclavian artery, close to the obliterated ductus arteriosus. Treatment involves resecting the stenosed aortic segment, and either fashioning an end-to-end anastomosis or placing a piece of prosthetic tubing between the two ends of aorta.

4 The principal risk is spinal ischaemia at the time of aortic cross-clamping, resulting in paralysis.

(See Chapter 9, *Lecture Notes on General Surgery.*)